Medical services and the hospitals in Britain 1860–1939

New Studies in Economic and Social History

Edited for the Economic History Society by
Michael Sanderson
University of East Anglia, Norwich

This series, specially commissioned by the Economic History Society of Great Britain, provides a guide to the current interpretations of the key themes of economic and social history in which advances have recently been made or in which there has been significant debate.

In recent times economic and social history has been one of the most flourishing areas of historical study. This has mirrored the increasing relevance of the economic and social sciences both in a student's choice of career and in forming a society at large more aware of the importance of these issues in their everyday lives. Moreover specialist interests in business, agricultural and welfare history, for example, have themselves burgeoned and there has been an increased interest in the economic development of the wider world. Stimulating as these scholarly developments have been for the specialist, the rapid advance of the subject and the quantity of new publications make it difficult for the reader to gain an overview of particular topics, let alone the whole field.

New Studies in Economic and Social History is intended for students and their teachers. It is designed to introduce them to fresh topics and to enable them to keep abreast of recent writing and debates. All the books in the series are written by a recognised authority in the subject, and the arguments and issues are set out in a critical but unpartisan fashion. The aim of the series is to survey the current state of scholarship, rather than to provide a set of prepackaged conclusions.

The series has been edited since its inception in 1968 by Professors M. W. Flinn, T. C. Smout and L. A. Clarkson, and is currently edited by Dr Michael Sanderson. From 1968 it was published by Macmillan as *Studies in Economic History*, and after 1974 as *Studies in Economic and Social History*. From 1995 *New Studies in Economic and Social History* is being published on behalf of the Economic History Society by Cambridge University Press. This new series includes some of the titles previously published by Macmillan as well as new titles, and reflects the ongoing development throughout the world of this rich seam of history.

For a full list of titles in print, please see the end of the book.

Medical services and the hospitals in Britain 1860–1939

Prepared for the Economic History Society by

Steven Cherry
University of East Anglia, Norwich

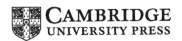

CAMBRIDGE
UNIVERSITY PRESS

CAMBRIDGE UNIVERSITY PRESS

Cambridge, New York, Melbourne, Madrid, Cape Town,
Singapore, São Paulo, Delhi, Tokyo, Mexico City

Cambridge University Press
The Edinburgh Building, Cambridge CB2 8RU, UK

Published in the United States of America by
Cambridge University Press, New York

www.cambridge.org
Information on this title: www.cambridge.org/9780521577847

First published 1996

A catalogue record for this publication is available from the British Library

Library of Congress Cataloguing in Publication data
Cherry, Steven.
Medical services and the hospitals in Britain 1860-1939 / prepared
for the Economic History Society by Steven Cherry.
p. cm. – (New studies in economic and social history)
Includes bibliography references and index.
ISBN 0 521 57126 X (he). – ISBN 0 521 57784 5 (pb)
1. Medicine – Great Britain – History – 19th century.
2. Medicine – Great Britain – History – 20th century.
I. Economic History Society. II. Title. III. Series.
R486.C48 1996
362.1′0941–dc20   95-50357 CIP

ISBN 978-0-521-57126-5 Hardback
ISBN 978-0-521-57784-7 Paperback

Contents

Tables

Note on references

References in the text within square brackets relate to the numbered items in the Bibliography, followed, where necessary, by the page numbers in italics, for example [5:27].

1
Contexts

(i) Introduction

This booklet examines the development of medical services and arrangements for health care in Britain from the mid-nineteenth century until the eve of World War Two. It follows the survey in this series by Roy Porter and anticipates a third study by Virginia Berridge [8]. In the period reviewed a number of vital changes occurred. Mortality rates fell, with major variations according to age, social class and region, and the contribution of medical effort to this decline remains controversial. Recognised causes of mortality and morbidity also changed, with the concept of epidemiological transition, the broad replacement of infectious diseases by chronic and degenerative illnesses, a useful if not totally adequate guide [76]. Perceptions of sickness and health, as well as formal medicine and health care systems, were increasingly influenced by scientific and professional opinion. Bolstered by advances in knowledge and techniques, by its own organisational successes and with some assistance from state legislation, the medical profession expanded and enhanced its economic and social standing.

For most people basic standards of sanitation were improving over the last quarter of the nineteenth century and, it was now assumed, the development of personalised services could make an increasing contribution to health levels. The workings of the medical marketplace, the poor law, local authorities, voluntary institutions and the state each had a role to play, though respective weightings and patterns of combination varied over time. Hospital treatments, courtesy of medical research, specialisation and nursing reform took on new public esteem. If the teaching hospital represented the pinnacle of medical achievement, specialist and general facilities expanded throughout the voluntary hospitals sector, with a rural element in the shape of cottage hospitals. Poor law medical provision also improved and, given appropriate political support and local government reorganisation, became part of a prototype public sector offering one model for a future national health service.

Best practice examples in public and voluntary sectors confirmed rapid progress, yet hospital and health surveys in the 1860s and late 1930s indicated variable provisions [112,121,125]. For the sick loss of income, fear of the doctor's fee or poor law institution often still accompanied the pain and uncertainties of illness. Medical practitioners were not that popular among the less wealthy and the approved societies, which administered the state health insurance scheme after 1911, even less so [88]. In the twentieth century the limits of voluntary effort and the insurance principle in health care were frequently discussed but less often acted upon. Financial restraints, ideological and professional interests dogged attempts to provide public sector alternatives [125]. Near-miraculous cures in the shape of sulphonamide drugs and technological breakthroughs such as radium therapy occurred alongside basic deficiencies, neglect and even discrimination at the close of the 1930s. Well before the test of World War Two the need for thoroughgoing reform was the one agreed point on the agenda of all interested in health care provision.

(ii) Medical history or social history of medicine?

This brief introduction suggests that the traditional concerns of medical history are too narrowly focused, though interpretation of the subject as by, for and primarily about doctors seems unduly harsh [12]. Yet there has been a strong identification of medicine with the practice of doctors or scientific researchers, particularly those heroic figures associated with its advancement. Medical progress is largely equated with the build up of a scientific body of knowledge and new techniques, with associated claims of objectivity, precision and increased effectiveness [27]. Cultural influences upon medical personnel or features affecting the outcome of medical practice, such as nutrition, are often ignored or assigned only peripheral roles. Similarly, the emergence of the medical profession and its exercise of power have been stressed in the context of decision making in hospital or asylum [20,25]. The medicalisation of aspects of social policy, such as the health of early twentieth-century schoolchildren, has also been a subject of controversy [102]. In turn, a distinctly anti-medical history has developed, focusing upon the inappropriate nature of medical intervention in, say, mental illness, the treatment of depression or overwork. Yet medical dominance in the past can itself be overstated, with portrayal of patients as victims, cases or even specimens.

A broader approach to the history of medicine and health care has many precedents. The practice of preventive medicine was not subject to professional claims before the division between public health and scientific medicine from the mid-nineteenth century [8]. Early twentieth-century studies of health and welfare or interwar investigations into poverty and malnutrition preceded the discipline of social medicine in the early 1940s [5]. Seminal works in the 1950s and 1960s cast doubt upon the impact of medical effort and nursing reform, encouraging critical and evaluative research [58,28]. The contribution of income or diet relative to medical measures or opinion resurfaced in this period, in new debate concerning the causes of late nineteenth-century mortality decline, infant mortality trends, the domestic impact of World War One and the 'healthy or hungry' 1930s.

Similarly with the delivery of medical services: not all sufferers became patients, nor were all healers doctors. Medical effort in its social context is a common theme in the social history of medicine, with the concerns of the sufferer and the role of lay care more fully acknowledged. Cultural influences which shaped medical knowledge and expertise may be traced via individual or communal experiences. Professionalism can be considered beyond possession of skills and specialist knowledge, with regard to questions of medical entrepreneurship, gender discrimination or the impact of interest groups on social policy formulation. The latter can be coupled with an assessment of life risks, or the meeting of social need vis-à-vis other objectives, such as social control.

With a more comprehensive approach some issues, such as

professionalisation or treatment of mental illness, have received more attention than others, such as occupational health or twentieth-century rural health care. Such imbalances cannot be remedied in this short survey but medical services and the hospitals are examined in a series of contexts. The remainder of this chapter considers the background of social policy and social risk. Chapter 2 outlines developments in medicine along with trends in mortality and morbidity, to see the likely scope of medical effort in relation to other influences. Chapter 3 considers the growth and consequences of professionalisation and reform in medicine and nursing. Service provision and patient access before World War One are outlined in chapter 4. This approach is extended to the interwar period in chapter 5, which also contrasts plans for coordination of services with practice and surveys facilities and opinion as to the direction of future reform. Finally, chapter 6 considers change in the funding of services and its consequences, returning to issues of accountability and control in health care.

(iii) Social policy and health care arrangements

It is not surprising that historians and others in the era of the Welfare State and the mixed economy were tempted to see past provision of health care and related services in terms of the development of social policy. The role of the state and policy formulation were central concerns and implicit in this approach was a steady progression from individual to collective provision. Such developments need not be socialistic, for themes of modernisation or of national interest suited equally well, and health care offered a particularly good example. In consequence of industrialisation and urbanisation, individuals could not reasonably be expected to provide for all their health needs, yet failure to do so posed a general health risk. Hence the gradual assumption by the state of responsibility for sanitary and other preventive measures, even if implementation devolved to local levels. Medical developments and increased awareness meant the continuation of this approach into a range of formal health services involving the poor law, local authorities, and arrangements with doctors and insurance companies.

In this evolutionary process there might be accelerations, occasioned by war or medical innovation, and periods of retrenchment, usually for financial reasons. There were arguments concerning motives, purposes and extent of reform, but consensus in two areas. One was that public services were extended, increasingly replacing private or philanthropic provision over the twentieth century. The route to the National Health Service was marked by legislative signposts. In its categorisation of the sick, the 1834 Poor Law Amendment Act had demonstrated awareness of the need for minimal, if less eligible, provision, while the 1848 Public Health Act set a more durable precedent for sanitary reform than earlier localised or emergency measures. Between the Sanitary Act of 1866 and the 1888 Local Government Act, the responsibilities of local authorities for sanitation and a range of basic health services, from support for salaried medical officers of health to provision of isolation hospitals, were delineated [79]. With the Metropolitan Poor Act of 1867 and provincial emulation, the treatment of sick paupers primarily under medical supervision was considered, opening the way to a 'hospitals branch of Poor Law administration' and, later, treatment of the non-pauperised sick [40].

A combination of philanthropic and local authority effort provided health visiting services in the early twentieth century, usually focused upon midwifery and infant welfare, though more attention fell upon the adult male oriented provisions of the 1911 National Insurance Act. This produced a state primary health care service offering sickness benefits and access to medical practitioners for 12.7 million people in 1913 [16 and chapter 4]. The scheme's critical flaws, lack of provision for the dependants of contributors or adequate hospital cover, were not remedied before World War Two and the introduction of an Emergency Medical Service. Neither the creation of a Ministry of Health in 1919 nor reforms associated with the 1929 Local Government Act offset these deficiencies. The ministry failed to coordinate existing arrangements and the 1929 legislation, facilitating local authority appropriation of poor law hospitals and the development of public hospital and health services, did little to guarantee improvements.

A second broad area of agreement concerns the impetus for reform. Workers or the poor, perhaps because of a lack of expertise or other priorities, allegedly displayed little interest in public health reform, so this was a matter for higher levels of policy making. There were tensions between the state and local authorities, or between civil servants and other bodies, notably the emergent medical profession. Aside from electing the occasional progressive councillor or passing conference resolutions, ordinary people figured to a very minor extent, though their interests were regularly evoked by social and medical reformers. With regard to health care, such views require considerable modification [chapter 6].

Features such as international economic and demographic – even racial – competitiveness loomed large in health and welfare reform [89]. British interest in national efficiency and fears of social deterioration by 1900 had continental parallels. French military and economic concern with lack of population growth stimulated infant and child welfare services, with municipal hospital and polyclinic provision geared also to TB and STD sufferers. Sickness and old age insurance provision, covering roughly eight million workers, followed by 1910. In Germany, compulsory sickness insurance from 1883 was part of 1880s legislation including industrial accident and old age provisions. One intention was to combat socialist ideas: the measures were aimed at urban workers in regular employment and involved graduated contributions and benefits. They applied to roughly one quarter of German workers, who paid for two thirds the cost of sickness insurance by 1914. The less organised, lowest paid or irregularly employed were mainly left to poor law style arrangements, again including TB treatments and dispensary facilities [89a].

In both countries levels of municipal hospital provision exceeded those in Britain until well into the twentieth century, but voluntary effort, works-based health care and insurance remained important. The USA provided a further contrast, for the late nineteenth-century expansion of health facilities was largely in hospital based personal treatment of acute illness, subject to maintenance charges and physician's fees. This represented a high cost form of treatment but patient pre-payment or insurance schemes were the popular response: charitable cases were a small minority and municipal, state or federal government efforts were limited to minimal services covering the poorest, particularly mothers and infants, and the mentally ill. Excepting a few social or medical reformers, self or family help with assistance from philanthropic bodies or via workplace schemes in a market environment was emphasised [99a].

Few historians now subscribe to a simple transition from individualism to collectivism in British health arrangements, or to social policy parallels with the medical history model outlined earlier. Some recent contributions can briefly be examined. It is more generally recognised that the formulation of policy might not mean rapid or thorough implementation and there is greater emphasis upon delivery and effectiveness of services [79,9]. Thomson rejects both etatist models and nostalgia for individualistic or neighbourly provision. His attempts to identify and measure amounts delivered rather than policies discussed in his work on the elderly led to conclusions that the emphasis upon individual, family or community resources varied over time, with the 1860s marking a lurch towards familial responsibilities [93]. Even including a generous assessment of poor law provision, such conclusions challenge the concept of transition from poor law to public hospitals in these years [39]. When developments in poor law facilities for the sick in the last third of the nineteenth century are set beside the promotion of self-help arrangements via friendly societies, provident dispensaries, sick clubs, hospital collections and fees, public sector-centred interpretations are diminished.

A simple transition from philanthropic to state funding in the pre-welfare state era should also be rejected. Philanthropic effort was always more complex than private donations from rich to poor. In health care especially there are strong solidaristic and public aspects to voluntary provision. A pooling of resources was often required to obtain medical expertise when necessary and to offset the consequences of illness upon income. Policy makers could accept the principle of government subsidies to charitable provision on cost effective grounds in obtaining expertise or services. There were also ideological aspects to forms of assistance which avoided public admission that care was the right of the poor rather than the gift of the rich [95]. Social control features might be detected in any charitable focus on the deserving poor, particularly curable and accident victims in hospitals or sufferers from occupational diseases, and these dovetailed neatly with industrial requirements [106,86]. The charitable 'case' in hospital was also very much under medical control, compared with the fee-paying domiciliary patient. Yet if professional influence increased over the late nineteenth and early twentieth centuries, it might partly be countered by the growing numbers of patients who had quasi-contractual arrangements via clubs or contributory schemes, or who were fee-payers, or who had a limited voice in hospital administration and funding [97,99].

These last features suggest grassroots, self-help approaches. From the viewpoint of social risk rather than social policy, Johnson has argued that the most common responses in the period 1870–1939 were private rather than public, collective not individualistic and local instead of national [104]. It is unnecessary to follow his classification of risk to appreciate that individuals could make strictly contractual arrangements or solidaristic ones, as in friendly societies, using a collective method to achieve goals of self sufficiency which had little to do with a proto-public sector. By the early 1900s more than 40 per cent of males aged over twenty years were friendly society members, but Johnson overstates his case in implying that the pre-national insurance population was comparatively well provided for. The low paid figured much less prominently and some nineteenth-century 'club' benefits offered minimal cash payments or treatments and also neglected contributors' dependants [87]. Allowing for other voluntary health care arrangements, the initial impact of state provision may have been exaggerated, however. Three quarters of those in the state insurance scheme were already sick club members and, though insured totals eventually rose over the interwar period, they represented 54 per cent of the adult population in 1936, compared with 47 per cent in 1914 [100,16].

For those at risk there was no guarantee of fundamentals to health such as adequate nutrition or housing. Contemporary investigation into interwar nutritional levels, for example, under the National Birthday Trust in south Wales or by MosH in north-east England, pinpointed the vulnerability of women and children, particularly in large families affected by unemployment [5]. Whatever the policy precedents inherent in poor law or sanitary institutions, the suggestion that an NHS for the poor was being created a century ahead of its time not only telescopes and oversimplifies the reform process, but understates social risks and their consequences [8]. If voluntary hospitals served the non-pauperised poor, they tended by rule to exclude small children and the infectious or mentally ill. In practice, they also offloaded chronic or incurable patients. Their reluctance to change this approach in the twentieth century made local authority provision even more important, as NHI arrangements did not cover hospital treatments on any significant scale. For the unprotected in health and insurance terms, the doctor's standard fee might be prohibitive. Well into the twentieth century chance and uncertainty were dominant factors, unless their requirements fell within the remit of special local authority provision, such as the 1919 Schools Medical Service. Geography also played a part; twentieth-century arrangements for the chronic sick or infectious in rural areas might be little better than the standards of the nineteenth-century poor law. Even those considered to be comfortably off might have insufficient resources for family practitioner or nursing home fees and yet be disqualified from entry into the NHI scheme or treatment without charges in a voluntary or poor law hospital by the 1920s. Thus life cycle and other risks to the individual were compounded by problems of access, type of illness and social status.

Two other features can be noted in considering individual risk. State social provision and medical professionalism did not signal the end of grassroots or lay effort. Treatment facilities arose via workplaces, communities or friendly societies and people relied upon self or family diagnosis and nosology (the classification of disease) before seeking other forms of care. It is not possible to elaborate on Porter's discussion of belief systems or experience of pain, but, in the context of appeals to study the sufferers' agenda, it is essential to note that people took care before they 'took physik' [92]. Decisions to visit the dispensary, purchase patent medicines, go to hospital or seek some possessor of specialist knowledge, be it herbalist, bone setter or doctor, involved assessment and use of what today is considered pre-primary care [1]. Perceptions of appropriate forms of treatment were influenced by income, kinship or community networks, religious belief (Methodist sects, Coffin-ites), or moral stances (anti-vivisection). Alternative systems such as homeopathy and herbalism or home-doctoring proved durable throughout the period, others, such as mesmerism or hydropathy, suggested faddism [9].

Such alternative forms of practice are not fully recorded, let alone quantified. If the influence of herbalism declined in this period, that of patent medicines increased. Reputation, cost, advertising and availability all figured in choices made and the absence of 'proper' medical services might be insufficient explanation. We can agree with Porter's general argument that all were affected by suffering. But not all were equally affected and some were better placed to complain, articulate or record their experiences, possibly producing distorted patterns of suffering. In the social history of medicine, as in the history of social policy, whilst noting 'who said what to whom and why', it is important also to utilise opportunities for 'measuring and assessing who got what from whom, when, how often and at what cost to giver, receiver or society at large' [93:357].

2
Medicine and its impact

Important changes in approaches to health care and improvements in medical services occurred after 1860. Greater control of life threatening illnesses, especially those associated with premature death, growth in formal health care systems, and improved medical knowledge all featured. The generalisation of such benefits is contentious, however, with one study referring to 'the irrelevant rise of scientific medicine' over much of this period [52:45].

Problems of definition, methodology and context influence any assessment of medical effort. If smallpox immunisation and hospital treatments had already reduced mortality before 1850, the former was an isolated medical triumph, while hospitals and their catchment areas were unrepresentative of medical effort or populations nationally [58, 53]. With hospital expansion, identification of functions or patients becomes more complex. Moreover, the isolation of strictly medical contributions from questions of diet, resistance to disease or ability of patients to withstand surgery is unrealistic given their interdependence in any assessment of life chances. Mortality rates offer a tempting but deceptive yardstick for medical impact even when accurately presented. Successful, rearguard medical effort may occur in periods of rising mortality. Medical interventions vital to individual sufferers and their dependants' interests may have little impact on overall trends. Even with cause of death established, mortality rates can be unreliable guides to patterns of illness, let alone health. And where health is interpreted as well-being, features such as social roles or relations of power also require consideration [5].

A simple relationship between medical effort and health levels cannot convincingly be statistically described. Instead, the approach adopted is to outline briefly some trends in mortality and information on morbidity. Medical improvement is considered, commenting on issues highlighted in optimistic accounts. Key arguments and recent research on the scope for medical contribution within wider influences on health are then examined.

(i) Trends in mortality and morbidity

Analysis of mortality trends is based on information compiled by the Registrars General for England and Wales from 1837 and for Scotland from 1855. Notification of cause of death was compulsory from the outset in Scotland but not until 1874 elsewhere. The inclusion of immediate and underlying causes, the addition of influenza and appendicitis as categories in 1891 and further changes in 1912 affected such data [60]. Underregistration of still births and illegitimate infant deaths was significant. Moreover, in the 1880s up to seven per cent of deaths in some northern towns were certified by persons not medically qualified. Identification of pulmonary TB, phthisis, bronchitis or pneumonia posed problems for doctors, as did the assignation of 'convulsions' as a nervous disorder or symptom of smallpox in infants. So did recognition of diphtheria, or diarrhoea as cause or feature in death. Deaths attributed to 'natural causes' in people regarded as elderly in the nineteenth century possibly masked industrial or degenerative diseases. If so, the predominance of infectious diseases then and the novelty of their replacement by chronic disorders in the twentieth century may be oversimplified.

Morbidity poses similar problems. National statistics were not compiled before 1945, apart from mainly infectious notifiable diseases. Data based on hospital, GP, friendly society or health insurance records may be unrepresentative. Improved access to medical facilities itself increased professional and public recognition of previously hidden illnesses [77]. Information can be ambiguous. For example, respiratory disease mortality generally fell in the late nineteenth century, but that from bronchitis and pneumonia rose. Between 1914 and 1918 civilian life expectancy rose, infant mortality fell, while dietary standards arguably increased, suggesting improved health levels [80]. Yet mortality

Table 2:1 Trends in crude death rates (CDR)and infant mortality
(IMR)1860–1939

CDR (per 1000 living)			IMR (per 1000 live births)		
England and Wales		Scotland	England and Wales		Scotland
1861–5	22.6	1860–2 21.5	1860–2	148	1860–4 120
1906–10	14.3	1910–12 15.1	1910–12	110	1910–14 109
1936–8	12.0	1930–2 13.4	1936–8	55	1935–8 77

Sources: B.R. Mitchell and P. Deane, *Abstract of British Historical Statistics*,
1962, pp. 34–7; M.W. Flinn [54], p. 382, p. 386.

among the elderly rose, the incidence of TB and VD increased and
war hardly promoted a sense of well-being [5]. In the 1930s
detailed local information indicating divergent health levels was
composited, providing less dispersal around national averages, the
whole allegedly mobilised for apologetic purposes [78].

There is little disagreement on broad mortality trends, sum-
marised in Table 2:1. In England and Wales stable mid-nine-
teenth-century death rates declined from the 1870s. Deceleration
by 1939 partly reflected an ageing population structure as birth
rates fell and life expectancy increased. In Scotland, CDR fell from
higher rates before the mid-nineteenth century and more slowly in
the twentieth. Mortality declined circa 1850 in the 5–34 year age
groups and among women aged 34–74 years, spreading to older
males, the aged, to young children and finally to infants by 1900
[63]. Whereas two thirds of those born 1838-54 reached the age of
20 and one half lived to 50 years, among those born 1910-12, four
fifths survived to 20 and one half beyond 60 years [64].

Throughout Britain mortality was lower in rural districts and in
suburbs compared with central urban areas, but the urban decline
was pronounced by 1900. Occupational variations actually
widened before overall improvements in the twentieth century
[51]. Violent death remained significant, fewer domestic or workplace accidents partly offset by road traffic casualties. Such features
help to explain lower longevity in men despite women enduring
the rigours of childbirth, lesser shares in family diets, greater
exposure to contagion through nursing the sick and defective
domestic environments. Dependants of males in high-mortality

occupations also suffered disproportionately and social class variations in deaths from diseases such as TB widened after 1900, as
poverty was expressed in mortality. By the 1930s death rates in
professional and business classes were respectively 13 per cent and
19 per cent below national averages for men and women, compared with 12 and 13 per cent above for unskilled male and female
workers [120].

Infant mortality rates averaged 150 per 1,000 live births in late
nineteenth-century England and Wales, though reductions in
suburban areas and in non-diarrhoeal deaths were already discern-
ible [65]. Death rates among 2–4 year olds declined from the
1870s. In Scotland, IMR was initially lower circa 1860 and
Glasgow had rates below most English cities, despite higher
illegitimacy levels. By 1911 IMR was broadly similar in all three
countries, falling more rapidly afterwards in England and Wales.
Maternal malnutrition and social class variation were common
features, but overcrowding was more extensive in Scotland and
local authority services less developed. Yet IMR among semi- and
unskilled workers in England and Wales in the early 1930s was 72,
compared with 39 in upper- and middle-class families. In Ply-
mouth, for example, subdistrict IMR varied between 16 and 109 in
1938 [5].

Comparing years 1848–54 with 1901 and 1971, McKeown
suggested that three quarters of the overall mortality decline
occurred through the reduction of infectious diseases. Table 2:2
summarises his evidence, giving examples from his classification
and noting in these the proportion of the overall (1848-1971)
reduction achieved by 1901 [58].

McKeown's interpretation is discussed in section (iii) but brief
comments concerning age groups, the situation in Scotland, the
interwar period and morbidity data are necessary. TB mortality
more than halved by 1900, though there were still 250,000
sufferers then and its incidence among unskilled workers was
double that in the upper and middle classes in the 1930s [9, 125].
Smallpox, scarlet fever and diphtheria figured among declining
airborne infections, but not bronchitis or pneumonia. Of water-
and food-borne diseases, cholera was virtually eliminated by 1900
but typhoid, not distinguished from typhus before 1869, remained
into the 1920s a more persistent threat. These features were similar

Table 2:2 Standardised death rates (per thousand pop.) by disease groups

	1848–54	1901	1971	% reduction 1848–1971 achieved before 1901
ALL AIRBORNE				
INFECTIONS (a)	*7.27*	*5.12*	*0.62*	*32*
e.g. respiratory TB	2.90	1.27	0.01	57
bronchitis, pneumonia,				
influenza	2.24	2.75	0.60	increase
scarlet fever, diphtheria	1.02	0.41	–	60
WATER and FOODBORNE				
INFECTION (b)	*3.66*	*1.93*	*0.04*	*46*
e.g. cholera, diarrhoea,				
dysentery	1.82	1.23	0.03	33
non-respiratory TB	0.75	0.54	–	28
typhoid, typhus	0.99	0.16	–	84
OTHER INFECTIOUS				
CONDITIONS (c)	*2.14*	*1.42*	*0.06*	*35*
e.g. convulsions, teething	1.32	0.64	–	51
ALL INFECTIONS				
(a+b+c) (1)	*12.97*	*8.47*	*0.71*	*37*
NON-INFECTIOUS				
CONDITIONS (2)	*8.89*	*8.49*	*4.70*	*10*
e.g. congenital defect,				
prematurity	1.25	1.37	0.32	increase
cerebrovascular disease	0.89	0.80	0.60	30
cardiovascular and				
rheumatic heart disease	0.70	1.67	1.77	increase
cancer	0.31	0.84	1.17	increase
STANDARDISED DR (1+2)	*21.86*	*16.96*	*5.38*	*30*

Source: adapted from T. McKeown [58], Tables 3:1–3:4, p54, 55, 58, 60

if slightly delayed in Scotland, though urban TB rates rose in the 1930s in unrelenting combination with poverty and overcrowding [78, 60].

Among childhood infections gastrointestinal diseases were prominent in infant mortality, as were the 21,000 deaths from 'teething' and convulsions in 1900. Congenital malformations and prematurity, amounting to three per cent of IMR in 1880, figured among deaths not attributable to micro organisms. Neonatal mortality (0–4 weeks) improved only slightly over the interwar years, but reduced post neonatal rates, with fewer deaths from diarrhoea, suggested better feeding and handling of babies by then. Comparing 1913 with 1935, there was a two thirds mortality reduction among 2–3 year olds while death rates among 3–5 year olds halved, reflecting the decline of measles, bronchitis, whooping cough and pneumonia [63,125]. Both diphtheria, with 50,000 cases annually in the 1930s, and TB still threatened older children.

With increased longevity and less infectious disease, so chronic and degenerative illnesses predominated among adults. After earlier underrecording and possibly a period of decline, heart disease and circulatory conditions such as thrombosis accounted for 22 per cent of deaths in Scotland and roughly one quarter of those in England in the 1930s [54,125]. Diagnosed in two per cent of deaths throughout Britain in the 1860s, the incidence of cancer, notably breast cancer, in adults aged over 35 years rose rapidly. Discovery of internal cancers saw a disproportionate male increase, with lung cancer prominent after 1930. These disease groups then accounted for most deaths among people aged over 60 years [9].

What of other illnesses? Wohl has described industrial diseases as a nineteenth-century way of life, noting their cumulative effect on mortality in men aged over 45 years and consequences for whole families [79]. Friendly society records indicate increased morbidity over the late nineteenth century, though life expectancy rose [110]. These relate to better-off workers, understating problems faced by women, children and the long term sick, even as access to health care improved. Interwar medical consultations suggest one fifth of illnesses linked to bronchitis, tonsillitis or colds, and one tenth each to influenza, rheumatism or lumbago, and injuries and accidents. Septic conditions, skin diseases and nervous disorders also featured among men, with women additionally affected by debility and neuralgia [125]. Given a supportive environment people could recover from many of these conditions, but the poorest, long term unemployed and dependants, and women with large families were most affected by income loss or inadequate services. Maternal mortality rates (MMR) rose in the late 1920s and early 1930s, with no improvement on 1900 levels until 1935, whilst further reductions in IMR dragged over the 1930s [56,78].

Variation in mortality and morbidity reductions suggested the need for wider economic and social improvement rather than purely medical efforts. Continuation of infectious diseases, if less fatally, similarly implied that public health improvements were less than decisive. Surviving infection and living longer, larger proportions of the late nineteenth-century population were vulnerable to degenerative and chronic diseases. Links between infectious and non-communicable diseases add new dynamics to the epidemiological transition and suggest that statistical presentations of mortality patterns may be too rigid. All underline the condition and behaviour of people in any assessment of the medical impact.

(ii) Developments in medicine

Medical achievements over the period were substantial. Whatever their claims in the past, doctors often operated on the basis of inadequate knowledge. Confronted by less obvious forms of illness, they might diagnose by inspection or touch and offer treatments which alleviated symptoms rather than underlying causes. By the late nineteenth century doctors could claim to understand disease processes more fully and justify medical interventions in terms of cure rates, prevention or management of disease or the alleviation of pain. Reviewing these developments, Sir George Newman (CMO to the Ministry of Health 1919–35) cited vaccination, anaesthesia, antisepsis and understanding of the causation of infectious disease as 'four great ideas' which helped to establish human control over natural forces and laid the basis for what today is understood as western bio medicine [11,123]. The emergence of a shared, universalised body of verifiable medical knowledge, developed and applied systematically by professionals and accepted by others as necessary and desirable, has often been presented in heroic or whiggish fashion by medical historians [23]. Here, some main features are outlined alongside indications of the need to qualify more optimistic interpretations.

By 1860 developments in pathological anatomy and the microscope had established a medical view of the body as comprising identifiable structures and organs which were affected by disease. While research and expertise in particular areas of the body were stimulated, such benefits were undermined if specialists paid insufficient attention to patients and their circumstances [15]. For example, neglect of occupational health in an increasingly scientific medical education led doctors to understate links between the working environment, the extent of chronic or degenerative illness and the role of both as a primary cause of death [76,77].

Understanding of the processes of infection dramatically improved over the second half of the nineteenth century. The idea of the body as a cellular mass, the identification of bacteria and the association of abnormal cell behaviour or the presence of invading micro organisms with disease made for systematic improvements in preventive medicine and surgery. Detection of specific bacilli allowed not only early diagnosis and more effective isolation procedures but also the opportunity for counter measures. For example, the discovery of the diphtheria bacillus in 1882 was followed in 1891 by development of an antitoxin which boosted body immune defences. Advances in bacteriology, associated with Pasteur and Koch, led to interventionist serum therapy against a major child killing disease. For many, this was indicative of the true scientific nature and benefit of late nineteenth-century medicine [2]. The growth of laboratory science, heavily utilising animal experimentation, and hospital-based clinical research occurred firstly and most notably in Germany and the USA. British emulation rested largely upon medical elites in the teaching hospitals and later upon public health laboratories, with 'Listerism' (see below) as its most significant late nineteenth-century achievement [21].

Dissemination of medical research and its application were not necessarily rapid, however, and the isolation of the TB bacillus, also in 1882, was not followed by immediate therapeutic gains. With new knowledge and isolation procedures, doctors were less likely to resort to dubious measures such as gum lancing, bleeding and emetics in the treatment of children suffering from fevers [9]. Yet gains in scientific medicine often occurred at the expense of earlier, lay emphases upon sanitary reform: serum therapy could be counterposed to wider environmental approaches in public health medicine, not least on grounds of cost or expediency [76].

By 1850 the introduction of anaesthetic agents provided relief from pain whilst extending the range and constructive aspects of surgery. Improved results were threatened by hospital infections, however. Antiseptic techniques developed by Lister from 1865 offered a partial solution but were not generally used before the late 1870s, not least because of the conservatism of surgeons themselves. Carbolic spraying during operations did not kill airborne micro organisms or compensate for inadequate hygiene precautions, exemplified in the surgeon's 'operating coat'. Some reduction in post-operative mortality also stemmed from improvements in the physical fabric of many hospitals [53]. In the 1880s the bacteria associated with surgical infections were identified along with phagocytes, those blood cells which resisted them. As all were vulnerable to antiseptic agents such as carbolic, the importance of absolute cleanliness in preventing infection was stressed. The surgeon's rubber gloves, gauze face mask, and sterilisation of instruments became part of aseptic procedures to create a sterile operating environment, but were not general before 1900. Laboratory aids to medicine and surgery also advanced with the introduction to Britain of X-ray equipment from 1896. In this example the rapid adoption of new technology was noteworthy, but an uprating of X-ray appliances and of user skills, critical to improved diagnosis, took longer.

Early twentieth-century medical services expanded and surgical procedures improved as a result of wartime experience, but the limits of purely medical approaches were emphasised by postwar influenza pandemics, which killed 150,000 people in Britain. It has been suggested that there were no major medical breakthroughs before the 1930s [42]. However, the use of salvarsan in the treatment of syphilis from 1910 represented the first cure of an acute infection. Bacillus Calmette-Guerin (BCG) immunisation against TB from 1924, the use of insulin in the management of diabetes after 1922 and kidney dialysis all originated in this period. Over the 1930s radium therapy, skin grafting techniques and blood transfusions were in their pioneer phases. Similarly the sulpha drugs, effective against specific infectious agents, were used in the treatment of puerperal fever from 1936 and pneumonia from 1938. The claims of scientific medicine were boosted by the anticipation that bacteristatics, chemical compounds which enfeebled target micro organisms, and antibiotics, the use of one form of bacteria (as in penicillin) to control others, would prove to be magic bullets in the medical armoury.

In most optimistic interpretations of medical developments the chief restrictive factor on further achievements was time. The generalisation of medical progress via professional skills, support services and the availability of hospital and other facilities for common benefit were also assumed. Such reasoning was challenged by contemporaries, including doctors. (see chapter 5). In the example of public health medicine, studies by Lewis suggest some loss of direction and purpose, despite overall expansion of services [23]. An initial focus upon dirt and sanitation until circa 1890 was replaced by more specialised attention on bacteriology, the role of isolation and disinfection before 1910, followed by interest in personal hygiene, health education and eventually services with a curative function by the 1930s. An optimistic interpretation of this pattern could emphasise the identification of problems and a responsive infilling with services, each reflecting contemporary medical knowledge and available resources. However, Lewis detects reluctance as well as difficulty on the part of medical officers in seeking further resources for health purposes and some narrowing of professional interests, despite an increased volume of knowledge in this area. One consequence was a crisis of specialism in relation to wartime planning and the concerns of social medicine by the 1940s.

(iii) The medical impact

McKeown's broad thesis assumes that long-term improvement in living and dietary standards, presumably reflecting market mechanisms, was responsible for most of the mortality decline [58]. This view is criticised by Szreter, who stresses the importance of social intervention, via local authority preventive measures and organisation of services, in the late nineteenth and early twentieth centuries [62]. Specifically, McKeown argued that scientific medicine could not have produced a decline in mortality rates before the late 1930s. The reduction of smallpox, limited success against diphtheria and a minor role for surgery represented its achievements. Improved nutrition was responsible for roughly half the reduction in mortality. Better sanitation made a smaller and later contribution, accounting for one quarter of the overall decline, with most of the remainder explained by changed virulence in micro organisms, notably associated with the decline in scarlet fever (Table 2:2 and [57]).

He reached these conclusions working back from mortality data, inferring ultimate cause of death and improving features by a process of elimination. This methodology requires accurate sources, correct inference and the acceptance of whatever variables remain after contenders have been eliminated. McKeown's information on diets does not match his analysis of causes of death and in 1880, for example, Registrar Generals Returns list 7.4 per cent of all deaths as unspecified and 4.9 per cent attributed to old age [52]. Moreover, his approach pays little attention to variations in population distribution, understating the importance and rapidity of mortality decline in urban areas by the close of the nineteenth century and the possible significance of earlier, pre-registration improvements [59]. He may have overstated the decline in respiratory TB, allegedly underway before general public health improvements and resulting from improved nutrition, paying less attention to geographic and sex differentials in TB mortality, which do not suggest monocausal explanations. Variations within McKeown's categories, for example increased mortality from pneumonia and influenza in the airborne disease group, and the separation of TB from non-infectious bronchitis or industrial illness, also pose problems.

Szreter's explanation of public health improvement by 1914 arising from social intervention deserves close attention. His approach recognises mortality variations and, notwithstanding debate on living standards, there was scope for sanitary, housing and factory reform and a possible medical contribution, via Medical Officers of Health. The timing of reform, as statute book legislation was applied at grassroots levels in the late nineteenth century, and its likely effectiveness, given predominantly urbanised populations, are both significant features. However, the uniformity of urban improvement is suspect, subject in reality to political and other interests requiring more than the passage of time or simple gestation of social investment [62,79]. Nor should McKeown's own recognition of such improvement go unrecorded [57, 58].

Any national impact on mortality rates from housing or factory reform or via improvements in atmospheric pollution by 1900 is also questionable. Guha has defended McKeown's emphasis upon diet, suggesting that even the most limited improvements or regular nutrition produced some benefit [55]. More damaging to Szreter's case, he argues that high morbidity rates indicate continuing exposure to disease. The latter was no indicator of urban improvement, whereas lower case fatalities probably reflected increased resistance levels, engendered by better diet or reduced virulence of micro organisms, or indeed successful medical efforts.

Taking a different approach, Mercer identifies smallpox, typhus and cholera as killers regardless of nutritional levels in the population [59]. Emphasising connections between infectious and non-communicable diseases he suggests, for example, that smallpox immunisation not only reduced fatalities but also side effects, such as reduced nutrient take-up and a susceptibility to TB, in survivors. Though smallpox vaccination decreased by 1900, effective monitoring and isolation procedures restricted new epidemic outbreaks in the early 1870s and 1890s. Each feature has a bearing upon the McKeown thesis; together, they undermine the validity of his disease-by-disease approach. Drug-based therapy for infectious diseases remained limited before the 1930s, but prevention or containment were important. Safe water supplies and adequate sewerage were critical in the reduction of cholera and typhoid, while mortality from typhus and typhoid fell by a factor of nine between 1860 and the late 1890s [9]. Doctors had little success in changing the course of infections once contracted and common illnesses such as measles continued to produce one in forty of all deaths, particularly among malnourished children, in the late nineteenth century.

The rapid decline of infant mortality in the early 1900s complicates arguments over environmental and nutritional influences. Szreter sees specific measures, including maternity services, safe milk supplies and hygienic food preparation as necessary to the fall in IMR and additional to other changes which had reduced general death rates [62]. Suggestions that infant mortality, particularly from diarrhoeal diseases, may not be a sensitive guide to improvements in the background environment before 1900 are not totally convincing, given imbalances between rural and urban rates.

Arguments that better nutrition and a reduced incidence of TB meant higher birth weights and stronger babies are contradicted by the high and unchanged incidence of congenital malformations and 'immaturity' in neonatal mortality well into the twentieth century. Deaths among older babies, aged 6-12 months, declined most, indicating that minimum standards set by the Board of Agriculture for cows' milk in 1901, the promotion of breastfeeding, improvements in dried milk powder and the rise of health visiting – whatever its social control functions – had positive results [9,67]. Gastro-intestinal illnesses, measles, whooping cough and TB were all reduced in infant mortality after 1910, reflecting background improvements now including reduced overcrowding and smaller family size.

A medical contribution to reduced infant mortality was limited and late. Roughly 70 per cent of births were attended by midwives by the 1870s but unchanged levels of infant and maternal mortality suggest that antisepsis and obstetrics were unproductive or nullified by interventionist methods in childbirth. Improved midwifery and other services made some difference to IMR and MMR by the 1920s, even in the poorest areas where an ominous correlation between the two rates remained [56]. The introduction of food supplements for expectant mothers in the Rhondda in 1934 produced in 10,000 instances over the following thirty months a decline in MMR from over 6 to 1.6 per thousand live births, with a halving of stillbirths and neonatal mortality [70]. Such dramatic improvements were not generalised, however, and MMR averaged 6.7 throughout Scotland in the late 1920s [54]. Nevertheless, economic recovery does not adequately explain the sharp fall in MMR in England and Wales, from 4.1 in 1931–5 to 2.2 in 1940 [68,5]. Drugs to counter the sepsis which was formerly implicated in one third of maternal mortality and in abortion attempts, increased use of blood and plasma transfusions and further improvement in midwifery services from 1936 all contributed.

Were there other areas of medical impact? Hospital facilities improved from the 1860s, offering treatments beyond the scope of GP or informal care, though there are few attempts to assess these. An examination of Glasgow hospitals circa 1860–1910 suggests inadequate responses to TB and infectious diseases, though infectious cases were usually taken to hospital by 1910 [61]. Poor law hospitals held only a small proportion of those suffering from respiratory and chronic diseases and normally took only advanced TB cases, without prospect of cure. They provided limited care while general hospitals concentrated upon curable cases, including urgent referrals from dispensaries. In English industrial centres, hospital work focused upon surgery, particularly accident cases, but also debilitating illnesses [53]. Remedial surgery in cases of non- pulmonary TB, for example, may have amounted to one fifth of all operations by 1900 [2].

Hospitals with increased curative or reparative functions after 1860 and with higher proportions of GP-referred patients in the twentieth century possibly exerted containing effects on mortality rates. Information on acute bed numbers, bed occupancy rates and duration of inpatient treatments suggests that voluntary hospitals alone provided for roughly twelve inpatients per thousand population in 1911 and thirty by the 1930s [46]. A key issue is whether hospitals successfully treated a sufficient proportion of life threatening illnesses. Considerations of care, relief or pain reduction lie beyond statistical speculation, however. Hospital therapies were often temporary and their value restricted by the absence of services for discharged patients. Questions such as the increasing numbers and competence of medical and nursing staffs, service provision and popular access are discussed in later chapters.

What was the medical contribution to other services? Ironically, the emphasis on curative aspects in much of scientific medicine over the late nineteenth century sometimes diverted attention from broader influences on health. Preventive measures were essential in the reduction of infection on a longer term basis, even in populations not experiencing improvements in income or nutrition, for medical effort then cut with the grain. Without such measures its role was limited, as demonstrated in persistent mortality and morbidity differentials in the 1930s, an important qualification to views that nineteenth-century seeds of medical improvement flowered in the twentieth [8,62].

Medicine can also be considered in relation to individual contingent risks. Throughout this period, lay recognition of various 'spits', 'lungs', or 'rots' indicated occupational hazards. Survival chances and well-being varied enormously with work, with exposure to accident or long term illness and, for women, additional risks in childbearing or caring. Friendly society or trade union efforts to organise medical services did not always benefit the worst off or most exposed. Employers making medical provision for employees and their dependants before 1900 included the Post Office, most railway, gas and canal companies in addition to paternalistic or progressive concerns, such as Colmans or Brunner Mond [77]. Access to such services was something of a lottery and they often represented a cheap, part-ameliorative option, though their extent may be underestimated [86].

The importance of fertility control in reducing illegitimate births and attendant risks, or the threat of extra children to women's health, family incomes or overcrowding was also understated in medicine and social policy. Large family size had a bearing on exposure to illness, notably TB, and the risk of childhood infections becoming domestic tragedies. Inadequate maternal diet or ante-natal attention were often revealed in neonatal and maternal mortality. As with infant and child care, official and medical tendencies to deplore maternal or parental conduct often ignored questions of income or considerations of costs and likely outcomes of medical treatment, which figured so heavily in ordinary lives [9].

Life chances possibly reflected genetic considerations, for example in the incidence of some cancers. Relationships between infective agents and human hosts were also complex and variable. Thus, the decline in pulmonary TB could in part be linked to the loss of non-resistant individuals and the proliferation of the more resistant. Such interpretations do not diminish the importance of social intervention, however; questions of natural immunity in the case of TB are better understood in a long term and total context incorporating housing, diet, fresh air, the reduction of work-related and other forms of stress and so on [2]. Many doctors recognised this, but scientific medicine tended to look, with relatively little success before the 1930s, to the promotion of artificial immunity and serum therapy.

Finally the question of medical effort and the epidemiological transition, that is from infectious to chronic disease patterns, is worth comment [76]. Increased life expectancy, even if accompanied by new patterns of illness, suggests some successes for a combination of public health, standards of living and nutritional improvement. The extent of the transition may be exaggerated by insufficient recognition of chronic and industrial illness in the nineteenth century. If some forms of heart or circulatory disease, cancers and chronic illness reflected not only longevity but previous encounters with infection, then late nineteenth- and early twentieth-century aspects of the epidemiological transition were directly linked. Medical responses in this context made for particular difficulties. Heart disease or cancers were notoriously difficult to tackle. Chronic illnesses, often the product of ageing, work hazards or childbirth, might be managed, but medical interest or status here was limited. Commonplace defects in sight or hearing, or nose and throat infections, important in the context of well-being, began to be treated among children but less obviously in older age groups from the early twentieth century. Until then small children, along with women in childbirth, were probably most affected by adverse results from overzealous medical intervention. The replacement of folk or unorthodox medicine with bio medicine possibly increased such risks, though patent medicines taken in excess and more spectacular forms of unqualified doctoring were equally if not more harmful [9]. Either way, with the consolidation of scientific medicine and development of services more people came under its influence and, on balance, benefits.

3
Professionalisation and reform

Over the nineteenth and early twentieth centuries qualified doctors defined the basis of medical practice and began to monopolise it. They achieved self-regulation in training and conduct and secured public recognition for their contribution, as experts, to wider issues of health and welfare reform. The emergence and positive impact of the medical profession, supported by improving scientific knowledge and facilities and reformed nursing systems, seem fundamental in medical history. Professionalisation involved the downgrading of other forms of healing and the accumulation of powers over patients, however. Intra-professional rivalries and disputes with other carers seeking to emulate the doctors' example also featured. Although the consequences of medico politics can be exaggerated, professional aims and wider public health needs sometimes conflicted despite claims to objectivity or the public interest.

(i) Medical reform and influence

By the early nineteenth century the growing demand for improved medical attention resulted in medical practice which blurred traditional divisions between physician, surgeon and apothecary. Medical effort soon involved more than an elite reliant upon the patronage of the rich whilst the unqualified catered for the poor [24]. Surgeon-apothecaries, increasingly involved in midwifery, represented prototype general practitioners. By the early 1840s, almost 95 per cent of newly qualified doctors were members of the Royal College of Surgeons and holders of the Licence of the

Society of Apothecaries [2]. Their education was based increasingly upon university medical schools founded in London from the 1830s or provincial centres additional to Oxbridge and the Scottish cities by the 1860s [26].

The desire to improve market position, dissatisfaction with the elitism of the Royal Colleges and with undercutting from druggists and other lay healers fuelled demands for medical reform. Professional interests required limits on competition and charitable practice and differentiation of an orthodox medicine, stressing qualifications and expertise, from services based on the retailing of cures or drugs. Doctors might cultivate a good bedside manner or specialism with wealthy patients and uphold the goal of family doctoring, but most recognised that the poor could not afford full medical fees. One in six doctors in 1844 held poor law posts, with competition often used to lower conditions of service [18]. Consequently, while some advocated the medical rights of the poor others concentrated upon professional reform, attempting to establish a college of GPs in the 1840s.

The Medical Act of 1858 boosted the profession without resolving its internal tensions. The General Medical Council was responsible for the education and licensing of doctors, but uniform training or a single medical qualification were not achieved. Professional common ground centred on the medical register, exclusive to those who had passed the RCS, LSA or, from 1861, RCP examinations [26]. Those who feigned qualification could be prosecuted and alternative, implicitly lesser and unorthodox, forms of practice were detached though not prevented. Along with the threat of dismissal from the medical register, these provisions offered the public standards of competence and advanced professional interests by identifying qualified doctors for public posts and fee paying clients [24]. Under the GMC the replacement of medical education based upon apprenticeship and private anatomy class by university and hospital medical school rapidly accelerated. A five year minimum period of study and training, more closely supervised and culminating in hospital practice as clinical clerk to a physician or surgeon's dresser produced greater control of students by senior medical staffs. Through these members, domination of the GMC and the setting of examinations which defined the medical curricula the Royal Colleges' influence was

Table 3:1 Registered medical practitioners in Britain, 1861–1931

	Britain*	England and Wales**	Scotland	practitioners per 1,000 pop., England and Wales
1861		15,297	1,870	0.76
1871	20,084	16,292	1,762	0.72
1881		16,493	1,878	0.65
1886	25,998			
1891		19,037	2,595	0.66
1901	35,691	22,230	2,965	0.68
1911		23,469	3,228	0.65
1931		29,300	4,088	0.64

* includes registered practitioners in Ireland and overseas
** includes retired practitioners
Sources: Brand [13] p. 146, Brotherston [15] p. 99, Loudon [24] p. 309, PEP [125] p. 141. For Scotland, T. Ferguson, *Scottish Social Welfare 1864–1914*, 1958, p. 447.

enhanced. A conjoint Board of Examinations from 1884 and compulsory examinations in medicine, surgery and midwifery, required under the Medical Amendment Act of 1886, consolidated their position.

The profession's senior members thus largely controlled the processes which defined competence and regulated conduct. This might serve public interests, particularly in conjunction with improved qualifications. But the expense, duration and nature of medical education resulted in a range of entrants restricted in social class (a few scholarship or prize winners apart), discriminatory attitudes towards women and the perpetuation of established values [25]. Similarly, the combination of university and hospital environments with a medical elite, removed from wider economic and social conditions and the range of minor or common illnesses, was not the best preparation for general practice or good relations with the mass of less wealthy patients [125].

Table 3:1 indicates the growing numbers of qualified practitioners, though their ratio to population figures mask great variations (chapter 5). By 1931 there were 29,300 general practitioners in England and Wales and 4,088 in Scotland. Almost 22 per cent were located in London, with 66 per cent in the provinces and less than 14 per cent in Scotland by 1936. The table suggests an improving market position for qualified doctors, and the numbers so described after the 1858 act fell by almost 4,000 between the 1851 and 1861 censuses, but this is also a generalisation [9]. Few doctors could concentrate exclusively on family doctoring at commercial fees in the late nineteenth century. Even those GPs willing to provide some free treatment or to accept a percentage of unpaid medical bills required sources of income. Newly qualified entrants or those with unfashionable practices in poor areas were often unable to translate professional gains into material advantage. The expansion of the British Medical Association, formed in 1856, from 2,000 members in 1867 to 17,000 by 1898, only partly reflected their concerns. They did not control the BMA but supported its efforts to extend the range of medical care and looked to the professional image it defended.

Did professional and public interests coincide? The BMA was unenthusiastic about poor law salaried practice but campaigned for improved services in the 1860s, creating better conditions for patients and doctors. However, free doctoring or use of hospital facilities by those who could pay was a major professional concern and interpretations of public interest here reflected establishment views concerning self-help [42,48]. The BMA also resented club practice (chapter 4) and attempted to boycott worst paid posts. Failure here reflected some doctors' need of income, however basic, though others supplemented earnings or took posts to preclude potential rivals in their locality. In campaigns against advertising by medical aid societies and the producers of patent medicines in the 1890s the BMA aimed to counterpose family doctoring. If restrictive of consumer choice [100], it is noteworthy that the BMA saw itself as guardian of medical and public interests. These examples indicate neither professional unity nor monopoly over medical arrangements before 1900, but illustrate concerns over remuneration and the desire to extend medical control.

Established GPs with a local reputation and paying clientele were sometimes threatened by qualified specialists. Surgery was part of general practice and, with midwifery, an often claimed specialism. Over two thirds of GPs in 1886 were members of the RCS [15]. However, the association of medical specialisation with particular illnesses, areas of the body and hospital practice widened divisions with the GP's surgery or domiciliary attention. Some GPs doubled as 'GP specialists', for example as anaesthetists in smaller hospitals, but most were excluded from hospital work. They risked losing wealthier patients to hospital specialists who, acting initially as consultants, might then offer general services. GPs also feared the loss of working class patients to hospital outpatients departments.

Specialists' reputations rested upon tutelage of pupils, social connections or entrepreneurial activity as well as medical expertise. Many continued as family doctors to the wealthy but hospital appointments, particularly in teaching hospitals, became the specialists' hallmark. Concentration of research or skill brought professional gains and improved treatment standards, but not always without costs. Accelerated career development in voluntary special hospitals, often nakedly ambitious and at the expense of general medical knowledge or worldly experience, did not guarantee proficiency. Competition between medical schools meant increased emphasis upon merit in teaching appointments and gave specialists a new power base. In London teaching hospitals there was a 41 per cent increase in consultants between 1855 and 1889, while specialist numbers tripled [26]. Through their control of students, hospital bed allocations and influence as experts upon hospital governors, such doctors could determine policy in and beyond the teaching hospitals. Yet their selection of interesting cases for teaching purposes, demands for costly but often underused equipment and the proliferation of special clinics did not sit easily with general philanthropic objectives, and the very location of at least one London teaching hospital, St Thomas's, was partly determined by its convenience for consultants [48].

One solution to intra-professional conflict was the referral system. This simplified the demarcation of GP primary care and the specialist, hospital-based role of the consultant in the new medical orthodoxy. Extensive general practice became a possibility under the National Insurance Act of 1911. This secured the economic position and status of participating GPs providing primary care and responsible for certifying illness and eligibility for benefits (see chapter 4). However, GP involvement in cottage hospitals often indicated efforts to retain paying patients by extending their range of treatments [41]. An early emphasis upon inpatient contributions, the spread of the cottage hospital in suburbs and dormitory towns, the retention of one in five hospital beds by GPs and their performance of 2.5 million operations annually in the late 1930s suggest that descriptions of the GP as victim in the division of medical skills can be exaggerated [20]. Nevertheless, demarcation between the British GP and hospital consultant contrasted with the hospital-based specialisms of most American physicians, a relatively low status example of which was general practice.

Professional divisions in Britain also arose over the emergence of salaried medical officers of health with expanding concepts of preventive medicine. They had their own professional society, founded in 1877 and with 1,850 members by 1936. Medical superintendents and, after 1930 in cities such as Glasgow, district medical officers, operated in former poor law hospitals and re-placement municipal services. Both allegedly encroached upon general practice, though GPs were not routinely excluded from work in infant welfare centres or school medical services. Neither undermined the economic benefits most GPs derived from combi-nations of NHI panel work and private practice. Successfully disputing the level of capitation fees in 1923, the BMA was able to maintain these at nine shillings, the 1931 economy cuts apart, until World War Two. Almost three quarters of GPs obtained more than half their earnings from sources other than panel practice, and few other groups experienced an interwar rise of approximately one third in real incomes [16].

There were attempts to emulate the medical profession or to join it. The Society of Apothecaries was eclipsed by the Royal Colleges and hospital apothecaries were usually replaced by physicians' 'juniors'. Pharmacists had a professional training dating from 1841 and supportive legislation which specified their training and reserved some dispensing functions by 1868, but their association with trade and lay medicine, if economically rewarding, under-mined status and claims to expertise. Dentists achieved registration under the GMC with the Dentists Act of 1878 but could not bar unregistered practice or secure full professional status until 1921. Even then, they lacked access to a mass market as most people continued without treatment beyond extractions, which doctors could still perform.

The late nineteenth-century medical profession's attitude toward women entrants, to midwifery and nursing attracts considerable attention as its gender basis belies claims to objectivity. Over the eighteenth century practice by women in orthodox medicine was progressively restricted to midwifery, which was also eroded by family doctoring, the new and male specialism of obstetrics and the rise of the surgeon accoucheur by 1860. Midwifery, when presented as a largely unskilled package of services to poor women, lacked the status or levels of organisation seen among pharmacists or dentists. Attempts by middle class women to re-establish midwifery as a profession or to enter medicine produced sexist resistance, also based on fears for lucrative practice. Elizabeth Blackwell, by virtue of American qualifications (1849), Elizabeth Garrett, holding the LSA (1865) and Sophia Jex Blake (1876) were the first registered doctors. But from 1856 until 1881 women were successively blocked from access to medical schools, clinical instruction, examinations and medical licensing [25]. Their number then rose from 101 in 1891 and 477 in 1911 to 3,331 or roughly ten per cent of the profession by 1931 [9,125]. Most were engaged in local authority services or in women's or children's hospitals, vital but professionally less contested areas of work.

Though most doctors endorsed the subordinate female midwife, useful as a watcher or carer and enabling them to supervise more confinements, an independent profession was a threat. Attempts by the Female Medical Society to establish a Licentiate in Midwifery with medical registration in the 1860s were blocked. From 1881 the Midwives Institute renewed the campaign for professionalisation but Bills in 1890 and 1899 for the registration of midwives failed. The 1902 Midwives Act was a compromise. There was professional recognition, the requirement of three months professional training and the prohibition of new unqualified practice. But midwifery was not a self-regulatory profession and a Central Midwives Board, not the GMC, was the supervisory body. Qualified midwives practised privately, in conjunction with friendly societies or voluntary associations, but local authority services were stimulated by the 1907 Notification of Births Act and the 1918 Maternity and Child Welfare Act, while training grants were provided under the 1918 Midwives Act. A salaried local authority service was formally required by the Midwives Act of 1936, but midwifery remained a recognised but subordinated profession. The model was broadly replicated in the case of health visitors, required to qualify through a standard system of training and a central examining body from 1925 [32,6].

(ii) Nursing and its reform

Professionalisation figured prominently in attempts to redefine the nurse's role and improve standards. Hospital development required corresponding improvements in nursing, involving closer supervision of the sick on behalf of doctors. Demand from the wealthy for nursing and nursing homes also increased. Nursing offered a career structure, a rare opportunity for nineteenth-century women, but its potential was restricted by the low status accorded to basic care and the stance taken by doctors and some of the reformers themselves. A united profession with significant improvements for all involved in nursing was not achieved by 1939.

Traditionalist accounts stress the role of religious foundations in providing institutional care and promoting nursing reform. Thus, the Anglican sisterhood at St John's House provided nursing facilities at King's College hospital from 1856 and religion and philanthropy figured heavily in Liverpool's Brownlow Hill infirmary nurse training scheme from 1865. Florence Nightingale's interest in hospital and nursing reform exceeded the initial impact of the Nightingale School established at St Thomas's hospital in 1860, while her emphasis upon the practical and subordinate nature of nursing antagonised campaigners for professionalisation, restricted registration and self-regulation. In the ensuing 'nursing wars', protagonists such as Mrs Bedford Fenwick and the British Nurses Association stressed a successful three year training before nurse registration, but could only produce published lists of suitable nurses in the 1890s [36].

Most doctors considered nursing reform from their own requirements, rather than on organisational principles or enhanced nurse status. In London, with teaching hospitals and wealthy clientele, they often supported nurse registration. Yet this failed to address

Table 3:2 Nursing as an occupation 1881–1931

	Women nurses	All nurses	Trained/registered
1881	35,216		
1891	53,003		
1901	64,209	69,200	12,500
1911	77,055		
1921	110,039	122,051	25,000
1931		153,670	50,000

Sources: Maggs [33] p. 8, p. 9, p. 24, Abel Smith [28] p. 57, p. 117.

the overall shortage of nurses. In larger provincial hospitals matrons and doctors saw in nurse registration opportunities to establish training schools, check rising nursing costs and attract fees. Others feared the consequences of failure to achieve recognition as a training centre [32]. Qualified nurses also posed a threat to the rural GP, particularly with the growth of voluntary district nursing associations offering domiciliary and contract services to poor law and local authorities from the early 1890s.

There was wider support for a less qualified, less defined, less ambitious profession. Burdett's Official Nursing Directory in 1898 saw the nurse's position as 'subservient...there to carry out orders...not to decide what method of treatment is proper' [114:25]. The new model nurse was portrayed as single, conscientious, diligent on aspects of cleanliness and hospital economy [33]. Extensive use of unskilled or inappropriate care was clearly hazardous, particularly in the hospital environment, but it suited proponents of reform to emphasise dangers or describe existing practice in ways which denegrated working class women who often learned from experience of family illness or by observing other nurses and doctors.

Table 3:2 shows how nursing as an occupation expanded after the height of the Nightingale era, particularly in the early twentieth century, exceeding population growth rates. This suggests an intensification of care, though nursing shortage was endemic throughout the period. Under one third of nurses were hospital based in 1901 and most of the remainder nursed the wealthy. Some 400 voluntary district nursing associations existed by 1907 but their work for local authorities did not comprise a full domiciliary service and only 600 nurses were employed by the latter as health visitors by 1914. The proportion of trained nurses rose but remained low, one third of those described as nurses in the 1931 census were registered [34,28]. Some of the 10,000 mental nurses in 1900 held the certificate of the Medico Psychological Association, introduced in 1891. Almost all were male and men comprised roughly ten per cent of nurses in peacetime between 1901 and 1939.

Three quarters of the 16,000 other hospital nurses in 1901 were probationers, mostly in voluntary hospitals. In 1913 the ratio of voluntary to poor law hospital nurses was two to one, inverting the corresponding bed ratio. This situation was changing. The poor law in Scotland offered the first national nurse training system from 1885, though a survey of 50 English poor law infirmaries in the 1890s for *The Lancet* found only four with nursing arrangements comparable with voluntary hospitals. Usage of inmates as carers was restricted under trained supervision from 1897 and the number of poor law nurses rose from 3,000 to 7,600 between 1893 and 1913 [37,3]. Poor law and public sector nursing then expanded eightfold by 1937, outstripping a threefold rise in voluntary hospitals.

Contrasting with the vocational nursing model, Maggs's findings on nurse training in four provincial hospitals suggested young, inexperienced staffs with unchanged proportions of qualified nurses or of nurses to patients, job dissatisfaction and high staff turnover [34]. This echoed the Nightingale School's early experience, though Maggs's sources are limited and skewed towards poor law hospitals and his voluntary hospital example shows older, experienced nurses entering formal training. By 1900 training was systematic, with qualified hospital nurses as ward sisters rather than problematic 'Lady Pupils' [38]. Probationary nurses, delineated in ward duties and dormitory requirements from the domestic work of ward maids, themselves remained a source of cheap labour, paying training fees and receiving meagre payments only in their final year. The average hospital nurse received £17 annually plus maintenance for a 70-hour week in 1901 and could be hired out for private nursing by her hospital to boost fee income. As yet, nursing reform carried little financial reward.

After 1914 war demand for serving nurses aggravated the overall shortage. Large numbers of women with little experience and variable training took up nursing via charitable agencies such as the Red Cross and Voluntary Aid Detachments. Among established nurses the College of Nursing was formed in 1916 to defend standards and promote its own form of registration, endorsed by the Red Cross and some training schools. Meanwhile, the government's priority was the overall shortage. The background to the Nurse Registration Acts of 1919 included establishment of the Ministry of Health (see chapter 5) and anticipation that standardised nursing services would be required as health facilities improved [32]. A General Nursing Council, responsible for registration and supervision of nurse training, was founded in 1919 but this was no self-regulatory body and the sixteen of its twenty five members who were nurses lacked agreed views on professional development. All nurses in service since 1916 were entitled to register, a measure which excluded the VADS but included large numbers whose qualifications varied from one year's training to twenty years' service, while supplementary registration covered male, mental, fever and children's nurses.

From 1923 three years' training and examination success were prerequisites of nurse registration. Nationally recognised examinations and certificates from 1925 enhanced individual qualifications but many of the 1,500 nurse training schools were unreconstructed, not least since withdrawal of accreditation spelled financial disaster for the affected hospitals and produced local political pressure. Hospitals were allowed to group in order to meet training requirements in medical and surgical practice. Inadequate resources, lack of integration and reliance upon probationers for staffing, rather than training, featured in the voluntary sector, while the GNC had no jurisdiction over poor law institutions.

In traditionally lower status poor law nursing, overall expansion, more enlightened attitudes among some local authorities and a degree of trade unionism improved nurses' conditions [37]. For probationers in voluntary hospitals there was little progress. The RCN took an anti-trade union position and supported restrictions on probationer salaries as a means of attracting only the dedicated. Investigations by the Athlone Committee revealed that the 96 hour fortnight, achieved by London mental hospital nurses in 1918, was operative in only 21 per cent of local authority hospitals and a mere

12 per cent of voluntary hospitals in 1938 [28]. Between one third and one half of probationers failed to complete their training. Many joined the 20,000 or more 'basic nurses', unacceptable to the RCN, but eventually recognised as State Enrolled Nurses from 1943. It required new investigations by the Rushcliffe Committee, another wartime intensification of the nursing shortage and government subsidies before nurses obtained substantial improvements.

Nursing reform has been equated with progress and non-hospital or specialist nursing neglected. Faced with the medical profession and gender conflict, some advocates of restrictionism in nursing were no less elitist in their approach. Successful nurses had greater career opportunities, but their profession was subject to medical controls, particularly in hospital environments. Standards rose but there was a lack of investment in nursing and training was often a guise for cheap labour. An institutional life, interpreting patients' needs to doctors and carrying out medical instructions often resulted in unsympathetic care and a high turnover of nurse trainees. Given the nursing shortage, poor conditions of service reflected upon hospital and other authorities and a professionalism which failed to consider all nursing interests.

(iii) Consequences

Improved popular access to qualified practitioner services by 1939 facilitates the equation of medical professionalisation with public benefit. Yet self-enhancing and self regulatory aspects of medical professionalism had other consequences. In poor law and charity patients gratitude and deference were expected, but the doctors' professional authority and knowledge suggested new dimensions in public esteem. One resented experience among all but private patients was that 'a minute of the doctor's time was more valuable than an hour of the patient's' [70]. In larger hospitals the lack of communication with doctors, the interposition of nurses, loss of privacy, unsocial waking hours, waiting, noise and restrictions, all in the name of efficiency were common. Avoidance of such features was a recuperative aid in private patient treatments. In teaching hospitals attention upon 'the case' for instructive purposes further demeaned patients. Though apt, individualised considerations minimise patient influence and should not imply that only the modern doctor exhibited authoritarian traits [8]. Medical control was not conclusive, particularly where lay effort was collective and financial (chapter 6).

A wide literature on professional authority and medicalisation exists, much of it interpretive, and only brief examples can be given [25,99]. Figlio has stressed contrasts between observed life experiences and the approach of scientific medicine in diagnosis [98]. A fifteenfold increase in rates per thousand of those classified insane between 1807 and 1890 may reflect surges in mental illnesses or professional attempts to justify skills and purpose, the growth of asylums and desire to control a disorderly population by professional and social establishment alike [11]. Late nineteenth-century women, suffering from a new range of psychiatric illnesses grouped as hysteria, evidently required protection from the stresses of higher education or careers which might jeopardise their reproductive capacity [27]. Similarly their focus on maternal inefficiency as a contributory factor in infant mortality shaped the views of MosH on the nature of health visiting and infant welfare. Doctors were prominent in interpreting a range of issues including race, poverty, criminality, hereditary illness, alcoholism and sexual behaviour, the whole welded into alarmist speculations concerning national degeneration [21]. Eugenicist outlooks often underpinned schools medical services, which provided treatments and arguments for social reform, and also boosted medical incomes [102]. Medical research also linked malnutrition and ill health of mothers and children to defective mothering and housekeeping rather than poverty, as in south Wales in the 1920s, or underuse of available services, as in Scotland in the 1930s [107,5]. Finally, efforts by interwar doctors to reduce overprescribing and lax certification of illness have been cited as proof not only of their satisfaction with the NHI scheme but also of unsympathetic responses to occupational illnesses or injuries, underrepresented in medical education [17,77].

Medical claims to objectivity can be challenged, but professional influence and coherence are sometimes overstated. Compulsory vaccination against smallpox in the 1870s and 1880s and the inspection of women held solely responsible for sexually transmitted diseases under the Contagious Diseases Acts of 1866-86 represent examples of combined medical and state control. Yet medical policing was comparatively rare in Britain, indeed under-developed in the enforcement of factory legislation, though Scottish public health doctors had greater powers on sanitary matters. Intra professional rivalries arose over specialism, but also preventive medicine, the public sector and trade unionism. The BMA included 'unionists' and 'scientists' and roughly 5,000 doctors had joined the TUC-affiliated Medical Practitioners Union by 1936 [20,125].

The medical profession was able to define and regulate its work, gaining state support and public recognition of its expertise, but medico politics rarely determined social policy. With a secure market position consultants could consider remunerative salaried practice in the public sector. GPs had economic security but an uncertain medical role by the 1930s. The BMA sought good conditions for Medical Officers of Health though deprecating their salaried service and potentially competitive role. Such professional enhancement held no guarantee of improved public health measures, however. Though not solely responsible, MosH failed to provide a coherent philosophy for public health or the public sector which might have been expected from them, as professionals [22]. And while the BMA called for health reform, it saw improvement in terms of measures which also safeguarded the doctors' financial position. Professional tensions as well as influence thus carried into the shaping of the NHS.

4
Medical services 1860–1914

The convention of grouping medical services as primary or secondary only developed over the nineteenth century, partly out of demarcation within the medical profession. Medical attention was not restricted to qualified practitioners even after the 1858 Medical Act and self medication, family or neighbours continued to represent the first line of care. Between 1865 and 1905, for example, the number of retail outlets for patent medicines quadrupled, to 40,000 [1]. Smith's study furbishes evidence of good and bad practice among qualified doctors and other healers in the late nineteenth century [9]. Hospital outpatient departments often represented the point of contact with organised medicine, as GP referral procedures barely existed. Qualified medical attendance and better nursing are a useful test for improved standards in health care, however, and more people experienced both by 1914. New forms of payment for medical services emerged, notably around the insurance principle. Local authority provision extended to personalised and curative services alongside sanitary and preventive measures. Yet shortfall, omission, and lack of coordination featured in both emergent public and voluntary sectors.

(i) Club practice and the poor law

Although there was a 50 per cent increase in qualified medical practitioners between 1861 and 1891 (Table 3:1), great variation in levels and even trends of GP provision occurred. Census enumerators' books confirm the preponderance of doctors in the south east, with an average of 939 people per doctor in London and 726 in Brighton in 1886 [9]. In the West Riding of Yorkshire, comparable ratios deteriorated from 1,777 to 2,554 per doctor from 1851 to 1881. Provision was best in market towns with a middle class clientele, such as Wakefield, and least in heavily industrialised areas with poor populations, notably Bradford and Sheffield [71]. These figures say little about typical practice, other than the pull of market forces, as the poor were irregular consumers of doctors' services. However, forms of club practice, medical charity and the poor law increasingly used qualified practitioners as cheaper alternatives to the profession's preference for family doctoring.

Doctors might reduce fees or extend credit, reasoning that some remuneration was better than none. More patients and less time figured in this exercise and the doctor retained control, able to reject difficult chronic or infectious cases. Similar conditions applied in doctors' clubs, based upon weekly or monthly contributions. A third and more extensive system included works clubs, friendly societies and mutual aid societies. Works clubs, based on deductions from wages in collieries and other workplaces, especially in Scotland and the north east, might include dependants or hospital facilities by 1900. In these and friendly society schemes there were elements of lay control, with doctors usually employed on a part time basis, or for set fees, or on capitation allowances possibly including costs of medicines. Some friendly societies offered choice of doctor from an approved panel, but most included doctors' services in a range of benefits. Whatever difficulties this posed for the medical profession, the opportunity to secure medical cover and sickness benefit for as little as four shillings per year was attractive. Strictly commercial, medical aid societies offered limited facilities as a lure for life assurance business [100,20].

Free dispensaries originated in London and Scotland in the late eighteenth century, sometimes developing into modest general hospitals, as in East Anglia [82,97]. In larger dispensaries and friendly societies' medical institutes doctors were salaried and the separation of diagnosis and prescription from dispensing helped to limit early nineteenth century abuses such as bottle doctoring, which relied upon product sales rather than medical knowledge or skills. The cheapness and ubiquity of some medicines used was suspect, yet the dispensary's role has been undervalued. One modest example treated over 13 per cent of people in Stockton on Tees in 1861 [101]. From the mid-nineteenth century provident dispensaries became typical, reflecting new emphasis on self-help and professional campaigns to limit free medical attention. These dispensaries were often based on a penny per week contribution, with cover for dependants and occasional charity patients, though paupers were usually treated by arrangement with poor law guardians or relieving officers. In addition, branches of the BMA began to develop their own Public Medical Services on a wider area basis, the Norwich scheme involving half of local doctors by the early twentieth century, for example. The extent of club practice is now recognised. By 1900 over 4 million friendly-society members were eligible for medical care and 9 million for sickness benefit [90,100]. In Scotland friendly-society membership exceeded 280,000 by the early 1890s and cheap 'six penny' doctoring was extensive [4]. *The Lancet* estimated that one half to two thirds of urban populations obtained medical attention through sick clubs with half of doctors involved in contract practice [20]. Free dispensaries apart, these schemes did not treat those unable to contribute and hospital care was rarely included.

Poor law medical attention was initially subject to stigma and the claims of ratepayers. Requests for medical assistance were often delayed by fear of the workhouse and the service's own limitations. There were 2,680 poor law medical officers in 1850 and 3,458 outdoor officers alone by 1872, with subsequent growth mainly among workhouse and infirmary doctors [3]. After the 1858 Act qualified doctors were employed, but often on a part time basis and influenced by poor law relieving officers. Doctors, when required to pay for medicines from salaries or contract fees, or seeking renewal of their contracts, were unlikely to prescribe expensive drugs or dietary supplements. Competition between doctors was used to lower medical costs and relieving officers could refuse to pay for particular treatments. Both features were acknowledged by the new Local Government Board, whose largely lay inspectors supervised medical services after the 1871 Local Government Act [13]. The very appointment of doctors was an issue in the Scottish poor law. Despite enabling provision under 1845 reform legislation, nearly 10 per cent of parishes still relied upon payments to GPs for specific visits or services for paupers in the 1890s. Until then, poorhouse provision excluded the unemployed and, as in England and Wales, medical effort in rural areas often hinged upon a single individual or institution [4,81].

Poor law improvements were mainly urban, with the transition from workhouse sick ward to separate infirmary and then public hospital featuring strongly [69,40]. The number of poor law dispensaries, one model for public health centres, expanded in London from 6 to 44 between 1872 and 1886 [13]. Together, the 1867 Metropolitan Asylums Act and the 1883 Diseases Prevention Act provided for the institutionalised sick under exclusively medical supervision and without disenfranchisement virtually throughout London by the early twentieth century [127]. From the 1870s poor law MOs were likely to be full time and campaigns in the 1860s by their own association, the BMA and *The Lancet* for better provision had successes. However, the poor law dispensary movement was checked over the 1870s on grounds of cost, self help criteria and medical opposition to free services [25,13]. This reversal may have featured in the rise of provident dispensaries, noted above. Provincial emulation was limited; there were just nine poor law dispensaries in 1872 and only fifteen provincial centres where the 1867 legislation had been applied by 1910, while the part time MO remained the rule in rural areas [3]. Suggested improvements applied less directly to the outdoor sick, 119,000 in 1871, who still outnumbered indoor counterparts. Benefits such as nurse visiting were considered in the 1890s, however, and domiciliary care figured in the fourfold expansion of poor law nurses between 1872 and 1906. Finally, reforming zeal within poor law administration, associated with 1860s Presidents of the Poor Law Board, Charles Villiers and Gathorne Hardie, was not maintained. Poor law representatives among the majority of Commissioners considering reform between 1905 and 1909 still favoured their own distinct medical service and less eligibility was openly supported by J.S. Davy, head of the poor law division of the LGB [84].

(ii) Voluntary and poor law hospital provision

Since the eighteenth century voluntary hospitals had developed around the principles of charitable funding, free contribution of services by honorary medical staffs and free treatment for the appropriate, non-pauperised poor. Access to their facilities was not a matter of right. It was conditioned by a subscriber-recommendation principle requiring patients or their representatives, except in emergencies, to find subscribers and appeal for hospital attention. Philanthropy did not determine that hospitals were located in areas of greatest need and their admissions policies normally excluded the very young, pregnant women, and those deemed mentally disturbed, infectious or incurable. The pursuit of value and the proper objects of charity often meant emphasis upon cure rather than care, on surgery and restoration of labourers for work. However, evidence on the duration of inpatient treatments, sex composition or age distribution of patients is not conclusive [95,106]. If the rural poor lacked hospital access, the rich, normally treated at home, experienced few disadvantages; hospitals initially offered little beyond the domiciliary capabilities of a physician or surgeon.

There were hospitals in most provincial centres by 1850 but a novel feature was the specialist institution. Fever and maternity hospitals, fifteen of the latter established by the 1840s, were joined by facilities reflecting career and entrepreneurial interests of doctors. Specialist hospitals partly created their own demand. There were twenty eye hospitals by the 1830s, with institutions for the ear, nose and throat, the chest, skin diseases or mental illnesses generally preceding separate facilities for women and children. Early developments centred on London, where sixty specialist institutions existed in the early 1860s, but provincial and Scottish emulation was rapid [44,81]. Thus Great Ormond St Hospital for Children, opened in 1852, was followed by 37 other children's hospitals by 1888 [49].

Table 4:1 summarises hospital expansion in the period under study. In 1861 there were 230 voluntary hospitals with 14,800 beds, 5,200 of which were in London. Special hospitals provided roughly one eighth of beds, and almost one third of those in London [46]. The combined figure represents only 0.7 beds per thousand population and failure of the voluntary hospitals to match population expansion was one feature in the crisis atmosphere of the 1860s and 1870s. Overcrowding, the predominance of serious or urgent cases, and more ambitious surgery contributed

Table 4:1 Hospital bed provision c. 1860–1938

		England and Wales				Scotland	
	Voluntary	Poor law	(separate infirmary)	Local authority	Voluntary	Poor law	Public health
1861	14,800	50,000					
1891	29,500		(12,000)		6,000	4,500	1,500
1911	43,200	80,000	(41,000)	32,000	10,500	6,900	7,900
1921	56,600	84,000					
1938	87,200	56,000	(53,000)	67,000	14,100	5,600	15,400

Sources: England & Wales, Pinker [46] Tables I, p. 49 and XIV, p. 81.
Scotland, Levitt [91] Appendix 2, p. 308.

to increased hospital infections and mortality [53]. Investigations into these and constructional defects were undertaken by *The Builder* (1856), Nightingale's *Notes on Hospitals* (1859) and by Bristowe and Holmes for the Privy Council (1863) [112]. Bodies such as the Social Science Association also inquired into hospital buildings and finances, themes later developed by Henry Burdett and the Hospitals Association (1886) into a general attack on medical charity ([113], chapter 6).

This proliferation of information heralded considerable changes. Hospital rebuilding or extension provided a sound basis for new surgery and nursing reform and bed provision almost tripled between 1861 and 1911. Table 4:2 indicates changes in beds per thousand population ratios.

Bed capacity in the teaching hospitals grew by half between 1861

Table 4:2 Voluntary hospital beds per 1,000 population, England and Wales 1861–1921

	1861	1881	1911	1921
Teaching	0.26	0.25	0.23	0.25
General	0.33	0.52	0.60	0.72
Special	0.10	0.16	0.18	0.25
Unclassified	0.01	0.02	0.06	0.06
TOTAL	0.70	0.95	1.07	1.28

Source: Pinker [46] Table X, p. 69.

and 1911, barely matching population increases, though bed to population ratios of general and special hospitals almost doubled. Other developments included the formation of cottage hospitals. The term included ex-dispensaries with inpatient facilities, seen in parts of south west England, and hospitals established in smaller towns in addition to the classic 'village' hospitals founded at Cranleigh in 1859 and St Andrews in 1865 [42,81]. By 1875 there were 148 cottage hospitals and their number doubled over the next twenty years, providing one tenth of voluntary sector beds circa 1900 [41]. Their basic facilities were important for the rural poor, though most people were expected to contribute towards treatment costs. A second feature was the reduced duration of inpatient treatments, by roughly one third between 1861 and 1911 [46]. This reflected patient transfers but also increased emphasis upon the acute sick. Many patients were discharged prematurely and without follow-up care, a common fault before the NHS. Nursing and convalescent homes provided one bed per thousand population by 1911, only one third of which represented an extension of voluntary hospital care. Recovering patients were also transferred to outpatients' departments, which dealt with an ever widening clientele. Hospitals exaggerated their work, publicising attendance totals rather than treatments, but outpatient facilities, acting as a filter for inpatient admissions, were a major source of primary and emergency medical care.

Wide variations in provision remained, beyond rural and urban comparisons and not reflected in problems and features of the twelve London teaching hospitals [48]. Thus voluntary hospital bed provision in Glasgow was only half that in Edinburgh, respectively at 1.6 and 3.1 beds per thousand population, though both exceeded the English provincial average of 1.06 [4,46]. However, more of the larger hospitals were transformed into clinical research institutions and many historians have noted the imposition of technical over social criteria in hospital design and operation [1,9,45,95].

In poor law hospitals, standards and organisational principles, rather than growth, have attracted most attention though bed numbers rose by 30,000 between 1861 and 1911 (Table 4:1). Most were for the elderly and infirm and not medically classified, but separate infirmaries in Manchester and Liverpool each contained over 200 patients in specified wards by the 1840s [19]. Popular need, particularly among the chronic sick whose illnesses produced destitution, was extensive and shortly after the 1860s reforms one third of poor law infirmary entrants were non-paupers. Separate poor law hospitals also expanded, providing nearly 41,000 beds in 1911. London had 16,300 of these, with 10,000 more in Birmingham, Leeds, Liverpool, Manchester and Sheffield. In England the poor law offered 3.36 beds per thousand population by 1911, one third of these in separate hospitals recognised as nurse training centres [46,70].

The admission of non-pauper cases, a 36 per cent increase in indoor medical officers and a fourfold rise in nurses from 1872 to 1906, with an emphasis on nurse training from 1897, suggest better standards in poor law hospitals [3]. Improvements in Manchester were replicated in towns throughout the north west in the early 1900s and in London the best poor law hospitals were reckoned to rival voluntary institutions [45,48,70]. Yet the 300 rural infirmaries lacked surgical equipment and basic medical supplies and in 1901 only one fifth had appointed a superintendent nurse [3]. Scottish poorhouse provision also remained inadequate [91]. Such variations indicate the gulf between actual and potential in poor law facilities, often understated when social policy developments are highlighted.

(iii) Local authority provision

Proto-public sector hospitals did not exist before the 1860s and greater progress towards them occurred outside the poor law. The 1871 Local Government Act, which combined poor law and existing public health measures under the LGB, heralded wider implementation of national policy at local levels. Under the 1872 Public Health Act sanitary authorities were eligible for central grants to improve water supplies and sewerage. Such grants amounted to £11 million in total between 1842 and 1872, £22 million for the rest of the 1870s, the same in the 1880s and over £40 million in the 1890s [79]. A second indicator of improvement was the compulsory appointment of local medical officers of health, also under the 1872 Act. Their numbers rose from just 50 in 1872 to 828 in 1876 and 1,770 by 1900. As guardians of public health in areas defined by the 1875 Public Health Act, MosH burdens were heavy. Further responsibilities concerning workplace sanitary arrangements and the notification of industrial diseases were added by 1895, but the MoH's role remained that of watchdog, rather than guarantor of services.

However, local authorities were allowed to provide isolation hospital facilities under the 1866 Sanitary Act and could be required to do so by the new county councils, created under the 1888 Local Government Act, after the 1893 Isolation Hospitals Act. By then, GPs had to notify their MoH of infectious cases and local authorities could compel the isolation of such patients. These procedures increased in importance with advances in bacteriology and smallpox, scarlet fever and diphtheria epidemics between 1870 and 1893. Isolation was a community benefit which imposed costs upon the individual and a free service was required for maximum effect [45]. In London roughly one thousand poor law patients were isolated annually in the 1860s, compared with almost 14,000 public health status patients, over 70 per cent of all 'fever' cases, each year in the 1890s [40,48]. By 1911 local authority provision represented 17 per cent of hospital beds in England and Wales and 35 per cent in Scotland in 1914 [3]. Pioneer attempts to test and trace victims of TB and to provide milk supplies free of bovine TB were followed by the establishment of sanatoria. Yet just 14 of the 64 TB dispensaries were run by local authorities and one fifth of the 8,000 beds available in the 84 sanatoria in 1911 [2].

Maternity, infant and child welfare facilities were often linked with charitable provision. Concern with infant mortality and industrial efficiency fuelled fears of a 'degeneration' of the population as proportionately more children were born into the working class. MosH were not immune to such ideas and calls for maternal responsibility figured in their efforts to improve health awareness and personal hygiene. Midwifery facilities were often offered by dispensaries and club medicine and standards began to improve with the registration and training of new midwives under the 1902 Midwives Act. Voluntary health visiting, practised in parts of England and Scotland since the 1850s, developed as a local authority service in Manchester from the 1890s and targeted new mothers, as in Huddersfield from 1905. There are specific examples of women doctors employed as health visitors in Glasgow, the establishment of hospitals for babies, as in Manchester in 1914, and infant health centres, as in Finsbury, Sheffield and Leicester from 1907 [67,45]. Yet the general emphasis was upon advice rather than material aid. Perhaps 90 per cent of births took place in the home. Before the Notification of Birth Act in 1907 required inspection of the newborn, health visitors might be unaware of these; afterwards, services might still be inadequate or resented [62].

The purpose and nature of facilities for the mentally ill or handicapped is controversial, as much depends upon definitions of such illness and the powers exerted by custodians of normality. Two thirds of county authorities provided asylums before the 1845 Lunatic Asylum and Pauper Lunatics Act required this of counties and larger boroughs. Centralised supervision was extended by the 1845 Lunatics Act. These arrangements replaced private licensed madhouses, targeting sick paupers and the poor. Though some medical superintendents anticipated cures or benefits from refuge and adequate facilities, asylum patient numbers rose from 12,000 in 1850 to 27,000 in 1870, with the incurable, in effect, quarantined [73]. Asylums exceeding 2,000 beds became a feature, particularly in London and Lancashire. By 1900 there were over 100,000 asylum inmates, with others in workhouse infirmaries or boarded out in licensed houses [74]. Patient numbers in Scotland rose from 6,000 in 1860 to 16,700 in 1914, the proportion in poorhouses or boarding falling from roughly a half to one quarter [81]. Cost considerations loomed large in patient placements. Apart from the 10 per cent of asylum inmates for whom costs were recovered, charges were made to the poor law guardians. They minimised expenses, retaining 'quiet' cases, frequently the elderly or handicapped, and sending 'difficult' patients to the asylums [75]. In 1859 only 10 per cent of workhouses had separate insane wards while 45 per cent made no special arrangements for such patients, who comprised 4 per cent of the pauper population [69].

Late nineteenth-century reform was ambiguous. The 1890 Lunacy Act specified procedures for certification of patients in asylums. This stimulated office based, entrepreneurial psychiatry for the better off, but probably deterred the poor from seeking treatment [72]. Ironically, it coincided with early outpatient clinics, (as at Wakefield in 1890), the use of reception and observation wards in some asylums, and the establishment of psychiatric units in some Scottish hospitals, measures aiming to reduce the stigma surrounding mental illness. Expansion of the concept of 'moral insanity' to include lack of self-help or self control, similarly deterred voluntary patients. The 1913 Mental Deficiency Act, requiring a secure environment and appropriate training or help beyond the workhouse, has both humanitarian and harsh eugenicist interpretations [74]. Under it, local authority 'protection' for 7–16 year olds was applied to pregnant girls and young, unmarried mothers on poor relief, for example [125].

Local authority health initiatives often reflected civic pride and political objectives. As early as 1894 the London County Council envisaged coordinated public health services [48]. With Bradford, it was the first of 48 authorities organising school medical treatments before the 1907 Education (Administrative Provisions) Act's requirement of medical inspection [102]. Some MAB hospitals tackled all manner of cases, while Barry UDC had established a hospital specifically for non-infectious cases, including accident and acute surgery, in 1900 [70]. Absorption of poor law medical services by local authorities at county or borough level offered the basis for unified health services, not free but not stigmatised. This was the minority view on the Royal Commission on the Poor Law 1905–9. It reflected the Webbs' influence and was adopted as Labour Party policy in 1911 [94]. Such measures were endorsed by prominent medical opinion on national efficiency criteria or as a boost to preventive medicine. Government rejection guaranteed the prolongation of divisions within public services and with the voluntary sector and possibly restricted the horizons of preventive health care [7].

(iv) National Health Insurance

The 1911 National Insurance Act (Part One) was primarily concerned with reducing the pauperising effects of sickness, though its architect, Lloyd George, recognised the 'ambulance waggon' nature of the scheme and anticipated further developments. Government plans stopped well short of a coordinating

Ministry of Health, let alone a public health service, using the insurance principle to offset pauperism whilst improving access to medical facilities. The scheme was compulsory for manual workers aged between sixteen and seventy years and for other employees earning under £160 p.a. Weekly contributions entitled registration with a GP chosen from a listed panel, medical attendance, drugs and treatment. Other provision included sickness, disability and maternity benefits and, in theory, treatments for TB sufferers [84,89].

NHI administration by approved friendly societies and industrial insurance companies resembled club practice writ large, with compulsory elements. This aroused the antagonism of the BMA, which had not been consulted. The doctors accepted a public service restricted to low earners so as not to jeopardise private practice, but demanded representation in central and local administration and sufficient remuneration under the capitation system. In fact, they had the option of panel practice with the local insurance committees, while GP–patient registration excluded non-qualified or alternative practitioners. They secured medical control in treatments, representation on the insurance committees and the establishment of parallel area medical committees, leaving remuneration as the key issue [20]. A threatened boycott involving 26,000 doctors in January 1912 delayed full implementation of the scheme by twelve months but a compromise capitation fee produced a skeleton staff of enrolled GPs. This pressured the BMA into accepting what was, essentially, its victory [25].

The doctors' dispute occupied contemporaries and confirmed the influence of the BMA [13], but what did the 1911 Act mean for patient access? Most of the lowest paid enrolled with medical practitioners by 1912, at an average of roughly 850 per doctor, a considerable improvement [16]. Previous schemes, if extensive, were inflated by multiple policy holding and did not provide for the worst off [97]. Moreover, doctors' problems in treating adequately at annual rates of roughly four shillings were eased by better capitation rates, separate from treatment costs. Yet with private practice and up to 2,500 panel patients, many doctors confined consultations to the signing of sickness benefit notes and bottle medicine [2]. Such practices increased consumer suspicion of compulsory schemes at rates above pre-1911 levels. Exclusion of dependants was a major drawback; recourse to club practice or private treatment renewed questions of cost or availability and confirmed a place in twentieth-century medicine for poor law provision. Extensions to the GP service were also limited. Sanatoria facilities were inadequate, ophthalmic and dental services were offered only as discretionary additional benefits by some approved societies. Absence of hospital care undermined claims to specialism or a comprehensive service, notably for the seriously injured or acute sick. Important in extending personal health care, the NI scheme thus represented only the largest of uncoordinated health services [17]. It offered few links to preventive medicine, though patients could benefit from earlier consultations, or to local authority services or Board of Education arrangements for child welfare. The poor law was partly bypassed, not replaced and, as will be seen, further developments were less than Lloyd George's 1911 audiences may have envisaged.

More people obtained consultations, however brief, with qualified medical practitioners in 1910 than in 1860, a feature further enhanced by the 1911 Act. For those excluded, limited improvements in poor law and local authority provision occurred. Secondary care developed, though hospital referral systems remained obscure, particularly for patients. Specialisation and rural infilling figured in voluntary hospitals alongside uprated poor law infirmaries, albeit late in the nineteenth century, while non-stigmatised local authority facilities expanded. Whereas 8.3 per cent of all deaths occurred in these institutions in the late 1860s, the proportion rose to 16.2 per cent at the opening of the twentieth century, with both figures doubled in London [13]. Given greater resources and breadth of services the public sector could build on preventive medicine, incorporating earlier recognition of illness and forms of treatment rivalling the voluntary sector. Opponents and supporters of the 1909 Minority Report understood this. Coordination of existing services remained inadequate, however. A ministry of health was not yet accepted in principle, still less its role and powers. On these questions the legislation of 1911 offered only delay. Optimistic accounts of health care and access [13,2] thus impart a sense of social justice and policy changes not materially translated on a national scale by 1914 or even 1939.

5

Rival systems or integrated services?

With the experience of primary care services and developments in the hospitals prior to 1914, demands for the generalisation of improvements and access to more advanced forms of treatment increased. Inevitably, these had political and ideological dimensions beyond the technical and organisational problems arising and all involved in health care had particular interests, not least financial, to safeguard. Consequently, medical services in the interwar years offer many contrasts. Innovatory expansion in public and voluntary sectors accompanied proposals for their coordination, a task for the new Ministry of Health. Yet rivalries between these sectors, defence of professional and commercial interests, a generally discouraging economic environment and government reluctance to assume responsibility also featured. Achievements in terms of growth paralleled failures to secure comprehensive services or promote health levels in the wider context. Lastly, the planning, potential and best examples of services contrasted with lags in delivery or non-provision at grassroots levels: further grounds for argument or accusation.

(i) War and the Ministry of Health

The impact of World War One upon health levels and social policy is controversial and its short run consequences for medical and hospital services were mixed [66,80]. War effort stimulated concern over infant mortality and child care; in terms of mortality rates it was indeed more dangerous to be a baby than a soldier, and a proliferation of local authority clinics and health visiting services followed, part funded by central government. Systematic services were heralded by the Maternity and Child Welfare Act of 1918, though new employment opportunities for women probably had more general effects upon women's and children's health. On war fronts over 14,000 doctors participated in services reorganised around emergency treatments at casualty stations with referral and evacuation to hospital facilities appropriated by the War Ministry at home. These arrangements stimulated surgical practice and hygiene awareness [2]. Temporary hospital accommodation was constructed, and many workhouse infirmaries used by the War Office received new equipment and specialists along with better pay and conditions for their nursing staffs, with durable effects [3]. Troops and civilians were affected by the spread of TB and VD and government responses produced specific services. Treatment for TB among insured workers, a matter for County Councils under the 1913 Public Health Act, was universalised by the 1921 TB Act. Following the Royal Commission of 1913-16, the VD Act of 1917 encouraged local authority clinics, often attached to voluntary hospitals, offering free treatments. Advertising of spurious remedies was prohibited, but more obvious prophylactic measures were not publicised. With treatments under the Schools Medical Service beginning in 1919, new public health provision was significant, without indicating any eclipse of voluntary or insurance based services.

The creation of the Ministry of Health in January 1919 suggests direct government involvement in health care but this had few advocates and little material evidence. Supporters of the Poor Law Minority Report saw state effort as critical to improved standards and coordination of services. They advocated replacement of poor law by unified, county-based facilities, which voluntary hospitals might join, but not state control or nationalisation. If this implied competition with or replacement of the voluntary sector, the latter had no shortage of advocates. Most doctors opposed threats to private practice, the extension of state salaries or local authority control. Through specialisation many sought to capitalise upon rising public esteem and surgical skills acquired in wartime [44]. Voluntary hospitals offered one avenue and themselves utilised public support for a range of facilities beyond GP-orientated health insurance. Full employment, associated with war efforts, boosted the position of the approved societies. Uncommitted to a more comprehensive or specialised NHI scheme, they opposed the expansion of rival central or local authority services. Within the public sector, reformers such as Morant and Newman at the Board of Education advocated expansion of the Schools Medical Service. Newsholme and Lord Rhondda, respectively CMO and President of the LGB, supported the creation of a Ministry of Health covering all aspects, including a public hospital service [3]. Yet the LGB itself was defensive and suspicious of potential rivals.

Such conflicting interests hampered the Ministry of Reconstruction, further undermined by the Lloyd George government's tactical use of social reform and stress upon economy by 1920 [48,82]. When the Maclean Report suggested in 1918 the abolition of the poor law and transfer of its functions, including hospitals, to county and county borough councils, absence of central government resolve guaranteed compromise and a weak new ministry. Replacing the LGB, the Ministry of Health embraced an unreconstructed poor law and lacked administrative control over the NHI scheme. With restricted funds, Addison, as first Minister, could neither coordinate health services nor urge their expansion.

In 1919 Addison established a Consultative Council on medical and allied services to consider future provision. Its interim response, the Dawson Report of 1920, is notable for recommendations and aversions, rather than achievements. Improved medical knowledge and practice would be generalised through health centres with preventive and promotional roles, offering extensive services. Dawson's wartime experiences helped define the GP-staffed primary health centre, equipped with beds and basic surgical facilities, able to refer patients to a secondary hospital centre with special amenities and consultant staffs. However, the role ascribed to the GP, albeit in grouped practice, reworked family doctoring at community levels, bolstering the medical profession at the expense of existing public health services. State medicine and full time salaried work were discounted and there was only minority support for the principle of free treatment. The future of voluntary hospitals was not addressed and the nature of the coordinating body for proposed services was unclear [7,2]. None of this altered the positions of interest groups or mobilised significant new forces. Without supportive funding and faced with the voluntary hospitals' own financial crisis (chapter 6), the Dawson Report counted for little. For almost a decade even the planning of health services was reduced to piecemeal and inconclusive operations.

(ii) Panel practice and other basic options

Whatever its initial defects, the NHI scheme had growth potential and was the favoured option of the Scottish Medical Consultative Council and the medical profession [91]. It covered 13.3 million people by 1922 and 20.3 million by 1938, with women workers then comprising nearly one third of the total and young people aged 14-16 years newly admitted [111]. 16.7 million people in 1930 and 18.9 million in 1938 had formally enrolled on GP panels. However, the interwar average of between 900 and 1,000 patients per doctor was misleading [16]. With favourable capitation fees established after a dispute with the approved societies and the government in 1923, many doctors positively sought panel patients. A GP employing an assistant could have up to 4,000. Doctors could alternatively concentrate upon private patients, given a wealthy local clientele. Either approach meant pressure to reduce time spent with each panel patient, repeating a feature of nineteenth-century club practice. Though patients' visits doubled over the interwar years, only slightly more than half of panel patients actually saw their doctor in any one year in the mid 1930s [125].

The balancing of medical provision with profits in NHI administration became a major cause for public concern [88]. Approved societies offered as 'additional benefits' discretionary services beyond GP facilities. These included dental and ophthalmic treatments, technically available to 13.1 million people and 11.6 million respectively by 1936 but not providing adequate or routine care. Hospital facilities under these arrangements covered just 1.88 million [125]. Insurance companies' influence and intrusive efforts to attract commercial business from their official role were resented, but their role in health policy formulation was considerable. The 1924-6 Royal Commission on National Health Insurance recognised the value of earlier diagnosis and treatments under the panel system, but regretted variations in services and sought to introduce hospital and maternity care. Minority calls for municipal services were considered only as an eventuality; meanwhile a pooling of resources might fund improvements. Conservative attitudes among approved societies with surpluses in the mid 1920s and depletion of such funds afterwards belied such hopes. Central government provided little impetus or resources (chapter 6). With hospital insurance, there was no desire to disturb contributory schemes, particularly involving government expenditure, and approved societies were in a poor competitive position [97]. Health insurance could do little to promote the integration of services, especially the preventive. Assistance to 'bad risks', the chronic sick, elderly or economically inactive, was strictly limited. As the largest durable form of health provision, the NHI scheme remained a qualified success [17].

For fifteen million dependants of the insured and others excluded from NHI arrangements, alternatives were conditioned by income. Individual GPs sometimes provided sick clubs and over sixty area based, GP-run Public Medical Services covered more than 600,000 people in the mid 1930s. Arrangements for middle class clientele paralleled hospital private bed schemes, partly at the expense of the older nursing homes which still offered some 25,000 beds. Friendly society provision for dependants and juveniles at work contracted slightly over the interwar period. In Scotland and the north former works clubs reorientated upon GP cover for workers' families. Industrial welfare schemes also developed in 'new' industries, the replacement of paternalism with company welfare featuring strongly [86]. Productivity and company or national loyalty figured in industrial funding for research and services for sufferers from heart disease or rheumatism, though family values, eugenics concerns and moralism predominated in efforts to combat alcoholism [96,76].

One in ten married women were in paid employment and covered by the NHI scheme. For many others health care was inadequate, with thorough investigation officially avoided, not least to curtail demand for state services [23]. Local authority infant and maternity care under the 1918 Act was initially variable and frequently criticised by GPs as a rival to family doctoring, while many voluntary centres resembled shops for proprietary goods [70]. One in seven babies was born in hospital by 1927 rising to one in four by 1939. This was a matter of routine in London, where 80 per cent of women were delivered in hospital, a rare experience affecting 10 per cent in Norfolk. Rural provision for complicated deliveries often relied upon cottage hospital GPs or Public Assistance Infirmaries and involved critical delays. Even in better provided urban areas, tensions between hospital consultants and GP-staffed, LA-run maternity homes could affect services [45].

School medical services, operated by three quarters of local educational authorities before 1914, were often rudimentary and only 21 authorities provided for the two to five age group by the late 1930s [102]. Where children were referred for surgery or hospital treatments, cottage and smaller district hospitals could be taxed by more than routine operations. Tuberculous children and non-insured adults were assisted under the 1921 TB Act, the public share of the 22,500 available sanatoria beds rising to two thirds by 1939 [20]. Good diet, fresh air and rest were recognised, but surgery for TB remained extensive in the 1920s. Standards varied but the shortfall of accommodation, including that in PAIs, persisted.

Poor law medical officers and nurses provided more domiciliary care but for unmarried mothers, the children of workhouse inmates, for senile or infirm patients, institutionalised services often applied. Requirements of supervision and economy usually dictated this approach [3]. Understaffing remained chronic, but appropriation of services by Public Health Committees from 1930 resulted in improvements, notably in Glasgow and Birmingham, and extended coverage, as in Oxford or Nottingham. Local authorities had 50,000 available hospital beds in 1921, 80 per cent in largely outmoded infectious diseases institutions. Conversion into sanatoria or mental hospitals was possible but rural district facilities were unsuitable and the sheer number of responsible authorities, 1,400 in England and Wales and 1,900 in Scotland in 1929, blighted planned alternatives [47,91]. Where reorganisations occurred, Lewis sees the failure of MosH to develop community medicine as critical, while Webster notes their tendency to supervise services, rather than to investigate causes of ill health [22,78]. Health centre and positive health options were frustrated, Finsbury representing a rare LA-based polyclinic, and Peckham a unique variant upon GP family doctoring [105].

Of the 300 mental hospitals in 1930, 90 per cent were constructed before 1914. The war and overcrowding necessitated
more outpatient provisions, with voluntary attendance and LA
clinics encouraged under the Lunacy and Mental Treatments Act
of 1930. Yet in 1936 all but 5 per cent of 155,500 mental patients
in England and Wales were certified [125]. Almost 90 per cent
were rate-aided, with 80 per cent of Scotland's 21,000 patients still
designated paupers [4]. Elderly people lacking alternative accommodation became institutionalised; others, who might have benefitted, were placed under PAI provision. Special institutions for the
insane housed 14 per cent of poor law inmates in London in 1929,
but only 4 per cent in the provinces [3]. Similar variations occurred
among the 40,000 people classified as mentally retarded. Nearly
half were in LA accommodation, one quarter in voluntary institutions and the remainder in PAI or Public Health hospitals. Just two
thirds of LAs offered special facilities, while one fifth made no
systematic provision.

Working class families spent an average of 3 per cent of their
household expenditure on medicines and services additional to
NHI contributions in the 1930s [16]. This could indicate lack of
treatments or cheaper alternatives to GP medicine, enabling
poorer families to cope with sickness. Yet self-medication, increasingly using patent medicines, was rarely cheap while delay in
seeking appropriate medical care often proved costly and harmful.
Hospital outpatient departments or dispensaries remained
another option but free facilities were restricted. Though NHI
was extended, the needs of those excluded were undiminished
and all but the poorest hospital users still faced additional
charges.

(iii) Hospital provision

A feature of hospital provision in these years was voluntary sector
expansion. Bed numbers for the physically sick grew to 87,200 in
England and Wales and to 14,100 in Scotland by 1938 (Table
4:1). The duration of inpatient treatments fell by one quarter, to
average eighteen days, from 1921 to 1938. Beds per thousand
population ratios increased from 1.49 to 2.12 in these years, a

narrowed London and provincial differential reflected in respective 1938 ratios of 2.38 and 2.04. Bed occupancy rates rose from 79 per cent to 84 per cent, with greater concentration in teaching hospitals. Consequently, one in three hospital patients was treated in voluntary hospitals in 1938, compared with one in four between 1891 and 1921 or one in five in 1861 [46].

Expansion under financial uncertainty and institutional loyalty neither coordinated nor equilibrated services, however. In January 1921 the Cave Committee examined the voluntary hospitals' position. It proposed creation of a Voluntary Hospitals Commission with local coordinating committees. These would promote regional organisation around a central base hospital, providing specialist facilities, medical education and nurse training, supported by 100 bed district hospitals and a cottage hospital network. Though regionalisation became a watchword, these plans produced few results, as acknowledged by the 1923 Onslow Committee for the VHC, and contemporary publications [117,119,121].

Potential for service integration varied. Teaching hospitals averaged over 500 beds by 1938, but figured prominently among the 75 hospitals exceeding 200 beds, while 500 hospitals contained fewer than 100 beds. There were 600 cottage hospitals by 1934: suburban expansion doubled their under-utilised bed capacity to 10,000 in one decade. Accessibility of inpatient treatments was important, but these hospitals did not represent the health centres envisaged by Dawson. Their GP staffs were accused of over-ambitious and bad surgical work, though many used consultants and referred serious cases [41].

General hospitals were sometimes open to these criticisms and defects applied throughout the voluntary sector. Specialist facilities were not primarily located according to patient need, or were duplicated in general and teaching institutions, while expensive equipment was used ineffectively [124]. Intensive treatments for the acute sick contrasted sharply with lack of after care services. Assertions of independence by specific hospitals soured relations with public authorities and undermined inadequate efforts to assess overall area health needs. In Scotland there was greater role demarcation as most LA hospital beds were set aside for chronic sick, TB or infectious cases, but standards were often low [91].

For Manchester and Merseyside early municipalisation of poor law hospitals allowed access for voluntary hospital waiting list or post operative patients. In Birmingham, such 'transfers' averaged over 2,000 annually by the late 1920s. Voluntary hospitals simply dumping patients or expecting public sector complicity with their requests, as in London, risked rivalry and financially important LA contract work [48]. Limited collaboration also arose through hospital contributory schemes or the use of consultancy skills, normally by private patients [97]. As these indicated a changing clientele, expansion in the voluntary hospitals produced diminishing returns for the poorest.

Qualitative improvement, new functions and lost opportunities featured in the public hospitals. Bed provision increased by 4,000 to 176,000 or 4.29 per thousand population from 1921 to 1938. However, mixed institutional beds fell sharply while medically specific beds in separate hospital accommodation rose (Table 4:1). Expansion also occurred in public TB hospitals (from 7,000 to 16,000 beds) and maternity hospitals (from 2,500 to 6,500 beds). Larger poor law hospitals benefitted from public demand, changed medical personnel, new working methods and, sometimes, a positive commitment to public sector medicine. There was a 50 per cent increase in full time infirmary doctors between 1905 and 1923 in London, with consultant services and treatment of the acute sick a feature [3]. Public patients able to contribute to treatment costs and private patients, often with their own doctors, were admitted to improved poor law hospitals. Public facility support could be competitive: in Bradford, a 600 bed municipal general hospital, open to all, was established by 1922 [117 for 1923:*232*].

Nationally, 70 separate infirmaries provided 30 per cent of all poor law accommodation for the sick in 1925, with 75 per cent separate provision in London but under 30 per cent in the provinces. In rural areas three quarters of infirmary facilities were located in general institutions of fewer than 100 beds, physically tied to the workhouse and an older poor law mentality [3]. Such contrasts intensified over the 1930s and applied to other LA services reliant upon former poor law hospitals.

Local government reform in 1929 centred on the near breakdown of the poor law and control of higher spending authorities but offered some rationalisation of public health care. The poor law and its hospitals, along with the functions of former sanitary authorities, were transferred to county and county borough councils. Their new public health committees could appropriate hospitals, providing integrated services with a preventive dimension, with voluntary hospital cooperation encouraged by the offer of a consultative role. This enabling legislation exemplifies contrasts between potential policy development and material gains for service users. Appropriation of PAI accommodation and its more specialised use was essential to non-stigmatised public provision, which some saw as a challenge to the voluntary hospital system [125]. A conciliatory stance adopted by the London Voluntary Hospitals Commission as the LCC uprated appropriated hospitals from 1931 suggested this [48]. In the Manchester area consultants promoted coordinated hospital services to boost medical specialism and safeguard their position against salaried practice [45]. One fifth of poor law infirmaries, 109, were appropriated as general hospitals and 74 for special purposes by 1938. Success required suitable facilities, financial resources and political resolve, none of which was guaranteed, particularly in rural areas. County councils appropriated just 22 general hospitals, half by Middlesex and Surrey, compared with 49 CBC and 38 LCC appropriations (121 for 1938). In Scotland similar legislation produced little change outside Glasgow [91]. PAI provision continued as the lowest level of hospital facilities.

In 1935 the British Hospitals Association appointed Justice Sankey in an enquiry into strategies for the voluntary sector. Inadequate coordination was commonplace; 30 per cent of voluntary hospitals reported no developments under the 1929 Act, while 13 per cent failed even to respond. Sankey's 1937 Report suggested some pooling of resources for supply purchases and reduction of waiting lists but reiterated themes of regionalisation and public sector cooperation [99]. Financial aid from the Nuffield Provincial Hospitals Trust and the first of a series of regional hospital surveys in October 1939 suggested limited progress before preparations for Ministry of Health surveys and the wartime Emergency Hospitals Service. Left to their own devices, the voluntary hospitals achieved growth but skimped their share in the development of integrated services.

(iv) Taking stock

What conclusions can be drawn about health care by 1939? Ideological issues, particularly the state's role in medicine, were ever present, though often obscured by the practicalities of fund raising or appeasing local ratepayers [85]. Patient interests, choice of doctor, the individual role in voluntary effort, public accountability and the ending of stigma were regularly invoked, yet consumers of medical services had limited influence upon their organisation [7]. Optimistic assessments link expansion of facilities and qualitative improvements with reduced mortality, while vitality in the voluntary sector and public sector potential were noteworthy. Best practice examples confirmed reform processes while calls for national health services indicated a desire to consolidate and generalise improvements. More pessimistic views note persistent variation and poor coordination of facilities, gaps in provision, missed remedial opportunities and inadequate promotion of positive health.

All this applies in the hospitals. Voluntary hospitals claimed 1.39 million inpatient treatments in 1937, roughly 35 per thousand population, albeit with some double counting. Public hospitals could claim enhanced and more specific provision. Yet with two thirds of all hospital beds, the public sector had only one third of hospital medical staffs and one teaching hospital, Hammersmith LCC, to its credit. Hospital surveys suggested shortfall from national averages of 50 per cent for bed provision and nursing in some areas, with intra regional variations equally pronounced [47]. Urban and rural contrasts in both voluntary and public sectors were sharp, notwithstanding rural use of urban services. London still had twice as many public hospital beds per thousand population as the provinces in 1938 and four times more acute sick beds per thousand than in county council areas [46]. Moreover, the concept of the hospital as a supporting service for community care remained underdeveloped [43].

At primary care levels, insurance based and LA provision was uncoordinated and insufficient. GP family doctoring was not possible under NHI arrangements. Panel patients received less attention than private, while the long term unemployed and married women no longer working faced uncertainty over their entitlement to treatment. GP referral of routine cases to hospital outpatient departments ineffectively used facilities, wasting doctors' and patients' time. Economic interests also resulted in concentration of GPs in better off areas or the build up of panel numbers. Unevenness of GP provision can be overstated, but conclusions that few doctors had over 3,500 patients are hardly reassuring [108]. Those excluded from NHI arrangements found that free or low cost alternatives primarily reflected charitable or commercial interests or the specific, limited requirements of the state. The tangle of agencies and services did not promote positive health. Ministry of Health and local Medical Officers saw this and were in a position to exercise a coordinating role, including preventive care. Yet they were also aware of rivalries between voluntary and public services and within the medical profession. To publicise problems meant criticism of current services and demands for reform, but these were officially the guardians of public health [78].

However, there were signs of service coordination in many urban centres by the late 1930s and, accepting their limitations, the services were relatively cost-effective (chapter 6). In the USA, 4.1 per cent of Gross National Product was spent on health care in 1935, more than double that in Britain. A combination of philanthropic foundations, voluntary insurance, government subsidies and tax exemptions to American hospitals had produced insurance cover, often limited to accident and surgery, for well below half the adult population. Among those who could not afford to choose, state or municipal health facilities were far more restricted and less than 40 per cent of people had access to a physician [99a].

Awaiting an enlightened consensus to inform policy in Britain was time consuming and unrealistic. The PEP Report recognised that without adequate nutrition and accommodation personal or sickness services would be swamped [125]. It aimed to minimise ideological disputes, concentrating upon extended, GP-orientated services, regionally coordinated with the hospitals. BMA 1938 proposals for a health service for all, barring 10 per cent or so private patients, looked to extend the NHI scheme and maintain a pivotal role for the GP, again with regional coordination of public health and hospital services. The British Hospitals Association eventually recognised that regional services could not be integrated by allowing voluntary hospitals to select functions.

Many of these suggestions indicated attention to a proper splay of medical services, each representing a particular specialism or interest group, in each area over attempts to secure comprehensive and sustained improvement in popular health [99]. Agreement on regionalisation was hardly novel and was based upon opposition to socialised medicine. It ignored the fact that LAs were the major provider of services, the 1939 Cancer Act a latest example. Yet their potential for a coordinating role contrasted with a record of uneven provision and political or territorial rivalries. Regionalisation might compound these, even with compromises over methods of funding, the claims of professional expertise and public accountability. Thus, despite general recognition of the need for comprehensive, national health services, interest and ideology remained significant obstacles. With the threat of war the coordination of services, recognised as inadequate in peacetime, assumed new urgency but interwar experiences suggested that the state must take a decisive role.

6
Health care finance, accountability and control

The proliferation of health care services by 1939 was associated with changed patterns of funding. A detailed summation of mid-nineteenth century individual arrangements is not available but friendly society and provident facilities already represented additions to philanthropy and the poor law, soon followed by local authority services and amenities provided directly by or on behalf of the state. Yet themes of progression from philanthropy to public sector effort or from private to collective provision, raised in chapter 1, are too simplistic. New methods of funding also had implications for public perceptions of accountability and entitlement. These issues have attracted little attention compared with questions of professionalisation, or the ideological counterposing of public and voluntary provision as models for a national health service [6,11,99]. Popular interest in aspects of accountability and control in health care was not restricted to those able to afford private services.

(i) Public sector funding

As a service of last resort, poor law medicine was always subject to financial restraints. These eased slightly over the late nineteenth century, particularly with the growth of separate infirmaries and greater control within these by indoor medical officers. Poor law spending totalled £600 million between 1834 and 1908, a growing proportion associated with medical services. Including asylum inmates, the indoor pauper population amounted to seven or eight per thousand of total population over the period 1860–1914, though outdoor numbers were more than halved. Crowther suggests the rise in poor law loan debt, from 3 per cent of annual spending in 1869 to 8 per cent in the early twentieth century, reflected new building and improvements. Specific building and repair accounts averaged £2 million annually, or 8 per cent of all spending, from 1899 to 1914 and separate infirmary provision figured heavily, along with facilities such as nurses' homes [3]. Improved standards were reflected in a 125 per cent increase in costs per new bed comparing 1885–9 with 1900–5.

Despite attempts to check them (chapter 4) asylum charges for poor law patients rose from ten per cent of total spending in the 1860s and 1870s to 15 per cent between 1900 and 1919. Costs of drugs and medicines doubled from 1840 to 1881 and had almost doubled again by 1905, totalling £788,000, with roughly two thirds spent on indoor patients [127]. The efficacy of spending has been queried by Smith, citing the rise in administrative costs to 23 per cent of the 1904 total [9]. However, these included greater medical officer and especially nursing salary costs as services expanded. Recognising overall inadequacies and forms which did not materially assist its clientele, poor law spending trends suggest improvements in medical services, though totals mask continued variations and stigmatisation.

Local authority spending on sanitary improvement increased sharply over the third quarter of the nineteenth century, assisted by central grants, averaging £2 million annually in the 1870s and £4 million in the 1890s [79]. By 1892 expenditure on water supplies and sewerage accounted for over 40 per cent of the £200 million local government debt [9]. In the early twentieth century new health spending occurred, though this often involved contributions towards philanthropic effort rather than direct service provision. However, as early as 1905 the Metropolitan Asylums Board spent over £600,000 on public health arrangements additional to its principal institutions, the fever hospitals. Central government spending on social services rose in real and proportionate terms between the wars, though little of this funded peacetime health services compared with unemployed relief, housing or pensions [82]. Local authority spending was sustained at roughly 40 per cent of central, boosted by government contributions to TB, VD, maternity and child services. Under the 1929 Local Government Act these were replaced by a system of block grants which were mildly redistributive and allowed flexibility within overall limits provided local authorities initiated reform. Their rising health spending over the 1930s reflected the reallocation of former poor law hospital and medical salary costs to health categories after the 1929 Act, and low initial outlays. By 1934 public sector hospitals had a combined income of £19.6 million, greater than the voluntary hospitals, mainly from local rates. Patient contributions offset less than 10 per cent of general hospital and asylum costs, and approximately 3 per cent of costs in infectious disease, TB and other hospitals [125].

Surveys by J.R. and U.V. Hicks noted increases in health and particularly hospital spending to levels which they felt were pressurising local rates, a public parallel to the voluntary hospitals crisis. Economic difficulties, the requirements of housing and the unemployed affected but did not override tendencies among poorer spending authorities to uprate hospital provision or for those providing better facilities to maintain them [115]. Powell's reworking of this material recognises variations in provision but suggests positive attempts to correlate municipal hospital beds and medical staffs with perceived need [47]. Local politics, municipal pride, the attitude of the local MoH and state of voluntary facilities all featured. However, his emphasis upon hospital beds is not necessarily the best guide to quality of treatments and analysis of county borough councils omits the county councils, whose provisions were still more variable [108].

Financial problems in the national health insurance scheme began with its flat rate principle, as necessarily low contributions inevitably restricted the range of services and improvements. Commercial pressures among the approved societies resulted in a dozen of the largest industrial insurance concerns and friendly societies controlling 90 per cent of the scheme by the late 1930s. Combined with the effects of unemployment, poverty and sickness, this meant that roughly one third of all friendly societies went out of business between 1918 and 1936. As many were small and solidaristic in outlook NHI administration became more contractual and less accountable. The dominant concerns, building surplus funds in the early and mid 1920s, used these to offer additional benefits and attract customers. They were less interested in promoting general improvement, extending the scheme's coverage to dependants of contributors or to include hospital facilities. Nor did they cooperate in the pooling of resources, suggested as an interim measure by the Royal Commission on NHI 1924–6 (chapter 5). By the early 1930s the deteriorating economic situation produced a tightening of administrative arrangements in the face of unemployment and chronic sickness claims and even less interest in reform.

Central governments hardly set the approved societies an example. After introducing the Widows and Old Age Contributory Pensions Act in 1925, the Conservative government even tapped off health insurance funds for pensions purposes. Under the 1926 Economy Act, government contributions to the NHI scheme were cut from 22 per cent to 15 per cent of total costs of roughly £33 million [118 for December 1927]. Restrictions, for example on working women who had married and ceased work, rather than expansion became the theme in NHI coverage. Though Honigsbaum has stressed the retarding influence of the approved societies, Whiteside suggests their stance was reactive and understandable [103,111]. Governments in the 1930s, for financial and ideological reasons, sought to limit state involvement in medical effort.

Health service spending represented 1.1 per cent of gross national product in 1921 and 1.8 per cent in 1937, amounting then to £66 million. Direct government spending comprised only 4.6 per cent of this total, compared with 17 per cent under the NHI scheme, 17.4 per cent from voluntary sources and 61 per cent from local authorities [11]. The impact of voluntary effort is understated in these figures. Contributory schemes provided over £8 million, mostly for the hospitals, in 1936 while many people had to make arrangements for dependants outside NHI coverage. Other spending on private medical services is not included and expenditure solely on patent medicines was estimated at £30 million annually in the late 1930s [70]. Nevertheless, the importance of local rates and the role of local authorities in an era of voluntarism and government growth is clear in England and Wales, if less so in Scotland [91].

(ii) Changes in voluntary effort

Philanthropy and professional interest shaped the medical services available for the sick poor until the mid nineteenth century. Afterwards the growth of local authority provision was paralleled by changes in the voluntary sector, with the rise of self-help arrangements and a diminished role for philanthropic effort based on transfers from rich to poor. Often this involved a pooling of resources, seen by some historians as essentially collectivist, by others as the means to an individualistic end of self sufficiency. By the mid 1880s there were approximately 3.8 million friendly-society members and at least half had arrangements covering sickness benefit and treatment for their families. Not all the remainder had access to medical treatment, but many of the local societies were basically doctors' clubs and more informal variants of these may be underrecorded [90]. Though the financial resources involved are unknown, there were indicators of growth in this area. Doctors generally opposed free medical treatment and supported the objectives of self help. Their concern with the rise of club practice, some forms of provident dispensary, the upsurge of retail outlets and usage of patent medicines, suggests the strength of popular measures not engineered by the medical profession.

New sources of funding for the voluntary hospitals departed from the philanthropic approach. Part of the hospitals crisis of the 1860s was financial: the traditional workings of the subscriber-recommendation system were already under duress. The financial burden of the chronic sick was transferred to poor law and other local authorities, but treatment of the acute sick increasingly involved intensive nursing and greater levels of technical and research effort. Establishment costs for a cottage hospital in the 1870s were roughly £500 and the annual running costs for a voluntary general hospital were £2,000–3,000 in district and perhaps £10,000 in county institutions by the 1890s [41,97]. The London teaching hospitals were most affected, for the requirements of specialist departments and educational facilities, or the complexity of patient illnesses were compounded by features such as reduced rental income from depressed agricultural holdings. Their alleged lack of economy and competition for charitable resources produced demands for reform throughout the 1880s and

1890s and a limited allocation system from the Prince of Wales Hospital Fund, established in 1897 [48,109].

Direct charges to patients were limited to some London and cottage hospitals as yet, producing only 4 per cent of voluntary hospitals' ordinary income of roughly £3 million in 1911 [46,113]. More typical was the reworking of philanthropy. In Scottish hospitals free treatments continued on the basis of aggregate costs covered by an enlarged scale of workplace donations along with investment income. The introduction of Hospital Sunday in Birmingham in 1859 provided the model for congregational collections, though the devolution of philanthropic effort progressed more rapidly with the establishment of Hospital Saturdays from 1870. Workpeople's collection committees or independent workshop sections existed in at least 34 provincial centres by 1890 and were provided with limited rights of patient recommendation. This opened the door to quasi-insurance arrangements, with hospital facilities added to railway, pit or factory sick clubs [97].

Hospital almoners were used in the late nineteenth century to check charitable abuse, filter out patients to the poor law and, later, to assess patients for contributions. Other economy measures included the reduced use of medicines and drugs for outpatients, particularly after the NHI scheme became operative, more intensive bed use and shorter periods of inpatient treatment. Rising demand for hospital facilities was aggravated by a threefold increase in inpatient costs during World War One. Though hospitals were compensated by the War Office and Ministry of Pensions for immediate and rehabilitatory treatments of war casualties, a crisis atmosphere, intensified by the influenza pandemic of 1918-20, anticipated the withdrawal of central funding. This was the background to the Cave Committee and the establishment of the Voluntary Hospitals Commission in 1921 (chapter 5). In fact, government assistance was temporary and limited to £500,000. Only one quarter of this was allocated in the first year, 80 per cent of which went to London hospitals. Notwithstanding the reduction in general prices, the London hospitals experienced a tripling of real costs over the period 1913 to 1938 and most had chronic financial difficulties [48].

Few provincial hospitals were in debt, however. Many had annual surpluses and by 1930 had invested funds totalling £17.5

Table 6:1 Voluntary hospital income in 1930 by source (per cent)

	London	English provinces	Scotland
Gifts	38	52	40
Payments	27	16	7
Extras	11	9	27
Public authorities	7	8	4
Interest	17	13	21
Ordinary income	£3.4M	£6.1M	£0.9M

Combined income, all sources £15.6M. Source: Hospital Yearbook (119 for 1932)

million in England and Wales and £6.1 million in Scotland [119 for 1932]. Faced with a decline in traditional subscription income, most abolished the subscriber-recommendation system and introduced inpatient charges. Workplace and other collections were reworked as contributory schemes, with weekly payments exempting prospective patients from hospital charges. Most people took this opportunity to add the hospital facility missing from NHI arrangements and scheme membership, excluding dependants, reached 6.2 million in 1933 and 10.3 million by 1938 [90]. Membership levels were highest in provincial conurbations but well established in rural areas, notably Oxfordshire and East Anglia, less so in Scotland. In 1935 the schemes provided 27 per cent of provincial hospital income, with transfers between schemes agreed in most areas and the range of benefits extended to convalescent, ambulance and nursing facilities. Though coordination of local authority and voluntary hospitals was limited, the schemes' operations provided additional links and an increasing source of income for municipal hospitals. In 1937, 11 per cent of scheme income in Birmingham and 16 per cent on Merseyside passed to local public hospitals [126].

Voluntary hospitals received contract income for local authority services, notably for child, surgical obstetric, TB and VD patients (Table 6:1). They failed to obtain adequate reimbursement for treatment of NHI patients not in hospital contributory schemes or for road accident victims, as payments from approved societies and insurance companies rarely exceeded one per cent of hospital income. Invested funds remained important, though 'windfall' legacies and gifts were generally used for capital projects. The last significant area was patient charges. Private patients were admitted to cottage hospitals from the outset and to most voluntary, poor law or municipal hospitals by the 1920s. Private wards, blocks and insurance schemes rapidly followed, boosting hospital and consultant incomes but illustrating the changed objectives of the voluntary hospitals. Other patients' means were assessed by almoners who as yet had little of the social work role. As Table 6:1 shows, patient charges provided London voluntary hospitals with over one quarter of their income, but were less important elsewhere.

These figures mask the contributory schemes, presented within gift income, but suggest their greater impact in the provinces while illustrating overall variance in funding. Further development of the schemes and of patient payments over the 1930s offered a respite for many voluntary hospitals. Ultimately, extended access brought no guarantee of compensatory income, however, whilst higher contributory rates might deter participants. As various payments largely covered their operating costs and 'windfall' income did facilitate expansion, it may be argued that most voluntary hospitals were cost-effective, though this ignores questions of service improvement or integration or additional wartime demands.

(iii) Questions of accountability and control

Changes in the funding of hospital and medical services raised new issues of accountability and control. When philanthropic effort took the form of donations by the wealthy, 'objects' of charity, such as early nineteenth century hospital patients, had no more influence than did recipients of poor law services. The motives of donors varied, but they wielded considerable power. Voluntary hospital governors, for example, might specify or influence new projects or have a voice in medical staff appointments. They were guided by medical committees as professional expertise was recognised over the late nineteenth century, while the ending of subscriber-recommendation eased out the small donor, but the wishes of major benefactors required careful consideration. Within industrial welfare, medical research and services, financial contributors, including central government, aimed to promote efficiency or productivity, but also certain ideological or social viewpoints [76,85]. It does not follow that donor objectives actually modified recipient or participant behaviour, or that control mechanisms were the only forces in philanthropic effort [86]. Yet the promotion of self-help was a very public matter and late nineteenth-century opponents of free medical assistance made no secret of perceived class unitary aspects of cottage hospital building or provision for worker representatives on the committees of fund raising bodies.

Hospital Saturday and Sunday schemes aimed to mobilise small resources and promote self-help but, in London for example, tensions between the organisers of the respective schemes prevented their amalgamation [48]. Though philanthropic functions were always emphasised by hospital authorities, many contributors saw a contractual element in their weekly donations. Such views sharpened once contributory schemes were established. A Voluntary Hospitals Commission survey, published in 1923, found an equal division between independent schemes and those associated with a particular hospital, while direct trade union or friendly society involvement featured in 40 of 105 examined [117 for 1923:*274*]. Where contributory schemes were particularly well organised or the major source of funding, as in mining communities, their representatives expected a major role in the formulation of hospital policy. In a few areas there were fears that 'one class of the community' might assume control [124,126]. In practice, such representation was less prominent than medical committees or local establishment figures, but could make hospital authorities aware of the views of their paying membership. Consultants sometimes had to recognise that auxiliary services, ambulance and convalescent facilities could be as important as the latest example of medical technology. The Hospital Almoners Association survey, published in 1941, noted that contributory scheme patients tended to expect treatment as of right, while ratepayers in municipal hospitals also saw no element of favour. Trade union hostility to the almoner's role as investigator of means, rather than of health, was also reported. Assumptions concerning grateful patients, subordinate to hospital or medical authority and lacking any concept of entitlement thus require revision [116]. To increasing proportions of patients paying directly or via contributory schemes for treatment in voluntary or municipal hospitals by 1939 the publicised differences in forms of hospital organisation were probably less clear cut than in 1900.

It is now conventional to emphasise working class suspicion of impersonal or state social reform circa 1900. Based on poor law and compulsory insurance, this attitude was reinforced by means testing in public and voluntary sectors in the interwar years. The PEP Report of 1937 and Nuffield Reconstruction Survey of 1940 pointed to the popularity of hospital contributory schemes precisely because they were neither intrusive nor commercial [125,88]. Indicative of self-help traditions, such evidence does not imply antagonism to less bureaucratic local authority or state facilities, still less ideological opposition to them, as voluntarist advocates suggested [48]. Lay opinion often saw the state's role as benign, but was unclear as to positive objectives beyond themes of improvement and expansion. Over the 1930s local authority appropriation of poor law infirmaries was supported when it heralded an uprating of facilities and genuine public usage. The few examples of local authority public medical services, drawing upon contributions from those not covered by NHI, were also popular.

Evidence of ideological commitment to public sector health care is still more fragmentary. Hostility to the poor law widened support within the infant Labour Party for Fabian proposals concerning public medical services and figured in direct attempts at municipal provision before World War One. Yet labour movement involvement in the procurement and management of health care, alongside forms of self help and collaborative effort, was long established. The leading role of Labour local authorities, the formation of the Socialist Medical Association in 1930 and Labour's specific commitment to a socialised medical service from 1934 featured in the groundswell of support for a comprehensive health service [83,94]. Public opinion had not discounted an extension of NHI arrangements, however, and more technical arguments, for example over regionalisation as a step towards national services or an alternative to them, were not widely understood.

The formation of the NHS was no simple matter of meeting

social need, a reflection of consensus or an indicator of the influence of expertise upon social policy. Inadequacies in health care provision were generally recognised by the late 1930s, while wartime stresses and experience of the EMS from 1940 accelerated the coordination of health services and guaranteed state involvement. Changes in governments and policy, the role of the medical profession and Bevan's significance have attracted most attention and form part of Berridge's forthcoming study. Here, it should be noted that financial considerations went well beyond the question of doctors' remuneration. Initial efforts to extend NHI or to promote public and voluntary sector partnerships sought to restrict state expenditure. However, the voluntary hospitals' reliance upon wartime state subsidies and overall inability to mobilise additional resources undermined the claims of voluntarism and independence as organisational principles in health care provision. The local authority model was also largely discounted. Unevenness of services in the interwar years, rather than best practice examples, was a key consideration. Negotiations securing cooperation of the medical profession and involving nationalisation of the hospitals, further reduced the role of local authorities.

Organisation of the NHS was technologically based, heavily influenced by the medical profession and had few elements of grassroots participation. A Labour Minister of Health abandoned party objectives, such as the abolition of private medicine, and largely ignored the role of local health centres and traditions of local accountability. Minority discontent within the Labour Party or lack of popular outcry did not signify absence of public interest in health services, however. Sickness traditionally meant loss of income, insecurity, and physical or emotional pain. But people expected to encounter illness and, considering their resources, sought forms of medical expertise and remedy. Throughout the period surveyed there was broad support for the growth of medical services and improved treatments, whatever other professional or ideological objectives were served thereby. The prospect of NHS treatment at optimum standards, free at the point of use and collectively financed mainly from taxation, tapped long endorsed objectives of improvement and avoidance of stigma or subjugation. Heavy and unforeseen use of services also indicated extensive deprivation and shortcoming, whatever the improvements over the previous nine decades. Interestingly, other forms of contemporary welfare provision were more restrictive or represented responses to contingencies not seen as inevitable, such as unemployment or inadequate housing. This may help explain the particular appeal of health care, and the initial and enduring popularity of the NHS.

Select bibliography

1 General

[1] V. Berridge, 'Health and Medicine 1750–1950', in F.M.L. Thompson (ed.) The Cambridge Social History of Britain 1750–1950, 1990, Vol. III. , pp. 171–242. Good, concise and up to date coverage of a wide range of pertinent issues.

[2] F. Cartwright, A Social History of Medicine, 1977. Valuable, if slightly dated attempt to place medical developments in their social context.

[3] M.A. Crowther, The Workhouse System 1834–1929, 1981. Best coverage of its subject, with good section on poor law medical services.

[4] D. Hamilton, The Healers: A History of Medicine in Scotland, 1981. Wide ranging but patchy. See also [81] and [91] below.

[5] H. Jones, Health and Society in Twentieth Century Britain, 1994. Not comprehensive, but provides much needed focus on women and ethnic groups.

[6] A.Leathard, Health Care Provision: Past, Present and Future, 1990.

[7] J. Lewis, 'Providers, "Consumers", the State and the delivery of health care services in 20th century Britain', in A. Wear (ed.) Medicine in Society, 1992, pp. 317–345. Important essay addressing the recipient in health care provision.

[8] R. Porter, Disease, Medicine and Society in England 1550–1860, 1993. Excellent introduction, not least because of the author's own wide researches, and good bibliography.

[9] F.B. Smith, The People's Health 1830–1910, 1979. Thorough survey, strong on information and statistics, giving a sense of proportion in its coverage.

[10] A. Wear (ed.) Medicine in Society, Historical Essays, 1992. Good, explorative essays, those by Lewis [7] and Weindling [76] particularly relevant to this text.

[11] C. Webster (ed.), Caring for Health: History and Diversity, 1993.

Very useful text with noteworthy sections covering imperial questions, but spoonfed presentation.

[12]   J. Woodward and D. Richards (eds.) *Health Care and Popular Medicine in 19th century England,* 1977.

2 Medicine and the medical profession

[13]   J.L. Brand, *Doctors and the State,* Baltimore 1965

[14]   W.F. Bynum, S. Lock and R. Porter (eds.), *Medical Journals and Medical Knowledge,* 1992.

[15]   J. Brotherston, 'Evolution of Medical Practice', in Nuffield Provincial Hospitals Trust, *Medical History and Medical Care,* 1971, pp. 85–126. A clear, short survey.

[16]   A. Digby and N. Bosanquet, 'Doctors and Patients in an era of national health insurance and private practice 1913–38' in *Ec.H.R.* 41, 1, 1988, pp. 74–94. Statistical support for lay opinion concerning panel practice, but a profession-centred survey.

[17]   N.R. Eder, *National Health Insurance and the Medical Profession in Britain 1913–39,* New York 1982.

[18]   J.T. Hart, 'The BMJ, general practitioners and the state 1840–1990', in W.F. Bynum *et al.* [14], pp. 228–247. Entertaining account of the shifting concerns of the BMA.

[19]   R. Hodgkinson, *The Origins of the National Health Service: The Medical Services of the New Poor Law 1834–1871,* 1967.

[20]   F. Honigsbaum, *The Division in British Medicine,* 1979. Strong on medico- politics, but understates external influences shaping services.

[21]   C. Lawrence, *Medicine in the Making of Modern Britain,* 1994. New, interpretive text, with focus on issues concerning the suppliers of medical knowledge and services.

[22]   J. Lewis, *What Price Community Medicine? The Philosophy, Practice and Politics of Public Health since 1919,* 1986. Important treatment of the professionalisation of public health, suggesting shortcomings within the specialism itself.

[23]   J. Lewis, 'The Medical journals and the politics of public health 1918–90', in W.F.Bynum *et al.* [14], pp. 207–246.

[24]   I. Loudon, *Medical Care and the General Practitioner 1790–1850,* 1986. Key account, suggesting that 'general practice' developed earlier and more extensively than conventionally assumed.

[25]   N. Parry and J. Parry, *The Rise of the Medical Profession,* 1977.

[26]   M.J. Peterson, *The Medical Profession in mid Victorian London,* California 1978. Good on the reshaping of medical elites through specialisation, hospital teaching and entrepreneurial activity.

[27]   P. Wright and A. Treacher (eds.), *The Problem of Medical Knowl-*

edge, 1982. Questions the objectivity professed by scientific medicine.

3 Nursing

[28] B. Abel-Smith, *A History of the Nursing Profession*, 1960. Still valuable, though emphasis is upon hospital nursing.

[29] M. Baly, 'The Nightingale Nurses: the Myth and the Reality' in C.Maggs [33] pp. 33–59.

[30] M. Baly, *Nursing and Social Change*, 1980.

[31] C. Davies (ed.), *Rewriting Nursing history*, 1980.

[32] R. Dingwall, A.M. Rafferty and C. Webster, *Introduction to the Social History of Nursing*, 1988. A comprehensive account which lives up to its objectives.

[33] C. Maggs (ed.), *Nursing History, the State of the Art*, 1987. Uneven essays, some of which belie the title chosen.

[34] C. Maggs, 'Nurse Recruitment to Four Provincial hospitals 1881–1921', in C.Davies [31], pp. 18–40. Detailed, if narrowly based, research makes comparisons which debunk some mythology surrounding nursing reform.

[35] C. Maggs, *The Origins of General Nursing*, 1983.

[36] S. McGann, *The Battle of the Nurses*, 1992.

[37] R. White, *Social Change and the Development of the Nursing Profession: A Study of the Poor Law Nursing Service 1848–1948*, 1978. Useful study of a neglected but significant aspect of nursing history.

[38] K. Williams, 'From Sarah Gamp to Florence Nightingale: A critical study of hospital nursing systems from 1870 to 1897', in C.Davies [31] pp. 41–75. Examines the practicalities of hospital nursing and training during the build up of the 'nursing wars'.

4 Hospitals

[39] B. Abel-Smith, *The Hospitals*, 1964. Broad account and still a useful starting point, particularly on aspects of administration and service delivery.

[40] G.M. Ayers, *England's First State Hospitals and the Metropolitan Asylums Board 1867–1930*, 1971.

[41] S. Cherry, 'Change and Continuity in the Cottage Hospitals c. 1859–1948: The Experience in East Anglia', in *Medical Hist.*, 36, 1992, pp. 271–289.

[42] M. Emrys Roberts, *The Cottage Hospitals 1859–1990*, 1991. Useful account by a staunch supporter of cottage hospitals. See [41] to plug one regional gap in coverage.

[43] G. Godber, 'The Domesday Book of British Hospitals', in *Bulletin*

Soc. Hist. Medicine, 32, 1983, pp. 4–13. Fascinating account by a participant in the wartime hospital surveys.

[44]   L. Granshaw, 'Fame and Fortune by means of bricks and mortar: the Medical Profession and Specialist Hospitals in Britain 1800–1948', in L.Granshaw and R.Porter (eds.), *The Hospital in History*, 1989. The career and entrepreneurial activities presented by medical specialisation. See also [26].

[45]   J.V. Pickstone, *Medicine and Industrial Society*, 1985. Major study of developing hospital provision in Manchester and the north-west.

[46]   R.Pinker, *English Hospital Statistics, 1861–1938*, 1966. Companion to [39] above. Detailed information, but based on single year comparisons.

[47]   M. Powell, 'Hospital Provision before the N.H.S.; A Geographical Study of the 1945 Hospital Surveys', in *Soc. Hist. Medicine*, 5, 3, 1992, pp. 483–504.

[48]   G. Rivett, *The Development of the London Hospital System 1823–1982*, 1986. Thorough account and good comparator for [45] above. See also [109].

[49]   A. White Franklin, 'Children's Hospitals', in F.N.L. Poynter (ed), *The Evolution of Hospitals in Britain*, 1964, pp. 103–122.

[50]   Acton Society Trust, *Hospitals and the State*, 1955.

5 Mortality trends

[51]   M. Anderson, 'The Social Implications of Demographic Change' in F.M.L.Thompson (ed.) [1], Vol. I, pp. 1–70.

[52]   D.A. Coleman and J. Salt, *The British Population: patterns, trends and processes*, 1992.

[53]   S. Cherry, 'The Hospitals and Population Growth', Parts 1 and 2 in *Population Studies*, 34, 1980, 1 pp. 59–76 and 2, pp. 251–266. Response to McKeown [58a], suggesting a positive if limited role for the hospitals.

[54]   M.W. Flinn (ed.), *Scottish Population History*, 1977. Important reading for anglophiles. See also [4], [81] and [91].

[55]   S. Guha, 'The Importance of Social Intervention in England's Mortality Decline: The Evidence Reviewed', in *Soc. Hist. Medicine*, 7, 1, 1994, pp. 89–113 and Szreter's 'Reply', in *Soc. Hist. Medicine*, 7, 2, 1994, pp. 269–282. With [62], these contributions reflect renewed debate on the causes of mortality decline.

[56]   I. Loudon, 'On Maternal and Infant Mortality 1900–1960', in *Soc. Hist. Medicine*, 4, 1, 1991, pp. 29–73.Considers service provision alongside questions of diet and environment. See also [62], [67] and [78].

[57]   T. McKeown and R.G. Record, 'Reasons for the Decline of

Mortality in England and Wales during the 19th century', in *Population Studies*, 16, 1962–3.

[58] T. McKeown, *The Modern Rise of Population*, 1976. See also [58a] T. McKeown and R.G. Brown, 'Medical Evidence related to English Population change during the eighteenth century', in *Population Studies*, 9, 1955, pp. 285–307. Landmark contributions, increasingly criticised on methodology and interpretation of data. Some revisions are required (see [53], [59] and [62]) but the essential position is not yet refuted.

[59] A. Mercer, *Disease, Mortality and Population in Transition: epidemiological and demographic change in England since the 18th century as part of a global phenomenon*, 1990. Intriguing material on the consequences of disease processes. If fully substantiated this carries serious implications for McKeown's approach.

[60] R. Mitchison, *British Population Change Since 1860*, 1977.

[61] C. Pennington, 'Mortality and Medical Care in 19th century Glasgow', in *Medical Hist.*, 23, 1979, pp. 442–450.

[62] S. Szreter, 'The importance of social intervention in Britain's mortality decline c. 1850–1914', in *Soc.Hist.Medicine*, 1, 1, 1988, pp. 1–37. Important revision of McKeown, strong on the timing of mortality decline, but open to counter-criticism on morbidity patterns. See [55].

[63] N.L. Tranter, *Population and Society 1750–1940*, 1985.

[64] R.I. Woods, *The Population of Britain in the 19th century*, 1993. Good introduction but does not entirely supersede [60] above.

[65] R.I. Woods, P.A. Watterson and J.H. Woodward, 'The causes of rapid infant mortality decline in England and Wales, 1861–1921', parts 1 and 2, in *Population Studies* 42, 1988–9, pp. 343–366 and 43, pp. 113–132. Surveys a highly contested area. See also [56] and [67] for contributions and additional sources.

6 Health and morbidity

[66] L Bryder, 'The First World War: Healthy or Hungry?', in *History Workshop*, 24, 1987, pp. 141–155. See, with [80] below, as an introduction to debate on the impact of World War One on the British civilian population.

[67] C. Dyehouse, 'Working Class Mothers and Infant Mortality in England 1895–1914', in C. Webster (ed) *Biology, Medicine and Society 1840–1940*, 1981, pp. 73–98.

[68] D. Grundy, *Community Health Services*, 1974.

[69] R. Hodgkinson, 'Provision for Pauper Lunatics 1834–1871', in *Medical Hist.*, 10, 1966, pp. 138–154.

[70]   S. Leff, *The Health of the People*, 1950. Includes early critical assessment of health care from the recipient's viewpoint.

[71]   H. Marland and P. Swann, 'West Riding Medical Practice from 19th century census data', in *Bulletin Soc. Hist. Medicine*, 41, 1987, pp. 72–77.

[72]   A. Scull (ed.) *Madhouses, Mad-Doctors and Madmen*, 1981. Important critique of approaches to and treatment of mental illnesses, restated and updated in [73].

[73]   A. Scull, 'Museums of Madness Revisited', in *Soc. Hist. Med.*, 6, 1, 1993, pp. 3–25.

[74]   A. Walk, 'Mental Hospitals' in F.N.L. Poynter (ed.) *The Evolution of Hospitals in Britain*, 1964, pp. 123–146.

[75]   J. Walton, 'Lunacy and the Industrial Revolution', in *Journal of Social History*, 13, 1979, pp. 1–22. Shows how well-intentioned provision came under pressure in one institution.

[76]   P. Weindling, 'From infectious to chronic diseases: changing patterns of sickness in the 19th and 20th centuries', in A. Wear (ed.) *Medicine and Society*, 1992, pp. 303–316. Clear survey article dealing with the epidemiological transition.

[77]   P. Weindling. *The Social History of Occupational Health*, 1985. Valuable account, given the importance of working conditions as a factor in ill health and mortality.

[78]   C. Webster, 'Healthy or Hungry Thirties?', in *History Workshop*, 13, 1982, pp. 110–129. Key article taking a pessimistic position and casting doubt on the value of aggregated official data.

[79]   A. Wohl, *Endangered Lives: Public Health in Victorian Britain*, 1983. Important work which underpins interventionist arguments (see [62]) and makes for interesting comparisons with the alleged later role of public health doctors (see [22]).

[80]   J.M. Winter, *The Great War and the British People*, 1986. Optimistic account, emphasises full employment and improved nutrition in bolstering health levels.

7 Social risk and social provision

[81]   O. Checkland, *Philanthropy in Victorian Scotland*, 1980.

[82]   M.A. Crowther, *British Social Policy 1914–39*, 1988. Admirable survey, combining information and brevity.

[83]   R. Earwicker, 'The Emergence of a Medical Strategy in the Labour Movement 1906–1919', in *Bulletin Soc. Hist. Medicine*, 29, 1981, pp. 6–9.

[84]   D. Fraser, *The Evolution of the British Welfare State*, (2nd edn, 1984). Major text, but rather linear approach to social policy development. See also [93] and [104].

[85] M. Freeden, 'The Stranger at the Feast. Ideology and Public Policy in 20th century Britain', in *20th Century British History*, 1, 1, 1990, pp. 9–34. Covers a range of viewpoints, but begin with [82].

[86] R. Fitzgerald, *British Labour Management and Industrial Welfare 1846– 1939*, 1988.

[87] P.H. Gosden, *Self Help: Voluntary Associations in the 19th century*, 1973.

[88] J. Harris, 'Did British Workers Want the Welfare State?' in J. Winter, *The Working Class in Modern British History*, 1983, pp. 200–214. Suggests people knew what they did not want, viz. poor law-style provision and commercialism in welfare arrangements.

[89] R. Hay, *The Origins of the Liberal Welfare Reforms, 1906–14*, 2nd edn, 1983. Remains an important survey of a complex and contested area. See also [89a]. W.J. Mommsen (ed.), *The Emergence of the Welfare State in Britain and Germany 1850–1950*, 1981.

[90] P. Johnson, *Saving and Spending*, 1985. Notable examination of popular behaviour and a counterweight to social administrative views on welfare arrangements. See also [104].

[91] I. Levitt, *Poverty and Welfare in Scotland 1890–1948*, 1988. Reveals considerable differences in Scottish, vis-à-vis English arrangements.

[92] R. Porter, 'The Patient's View: Doing Medical History from Below', in *Theory and Society*, 14, 1985, pp. 175–198. Most valuable for broad approach and issues raised.

[93] D. Thomson, 'Welfare and the Historians', in L. Bonfield, R.M. Smith and K. Wrightson (eds.), *The World We Have Gained*, 1986, pp. 355–378. Revisionist essay stressing the pitfalls of a linear approach to the growth of state welfare.

[94] C. Webster, 'Labour and the N.H.S.', in N.Rupke (ed.), *Science, Politics and the Public Good*, 1988, pp. 184–202. Suggests the N.H.S. reflected Labour's positive involvement rather than an enlightened consensus. See also [83] and [99].

8 Social risk and medical provision

[95] J. Barry and C. Jones (eds.) *Medicine and Charity before the Welfare State*, 1991. Useful articles, see [96] and [106], and introduction.

[96] D. Cantor, 'The Aches of Industry. Philanthropy and Rheumatism in Interwar Britain' in Barry and Jones (eds.), [95] pp. 225–245.

[97] S. Cherry, 'Beyond National Health Insurance. The Voluntary hospitals and Hospital Contributory Schemes', in *Soc. Hist. Medicine*, 5, 1992, 4, pp. 455–482. Regional survey of changes in the voluntary hospital system and popular effort to supplement primary health care.

[98] K. Figlio, 'Chlorosis and Chronic Disease in Nineteenth Century Britain: The Social Construction of Somatic Illness in a Capitalist Society', in *Social History*, 3, 1978, pp. 167–197. See also [27].

[99] D.M.Fox, *Health Policies, Health Politics*, Princeton 1986. Important Anglo-US comparison, though its focus neglects some basic differences. See also [99a], O.W.Anderson, *Health Services in the U.S.*, Michigan, 1985, for US information but note its over-optimistic assessment.

[100] D.G.Green, *Working Class Patients and the Medical Establishment*, 1985. Critique of the medical profession, less convincing on the benefits of market forces for those in no position to choose, and little on hospitals.

[101] R.P. Hastings, 'A nineteenth century dispensary at work', in *Local History*, 10, 1973, 5. Short, sharp and very useful.

[102] H. Hendrick, 'Child Labour, Medical Capital and the School Medical Service c1890–1918', in R.Cooter, (ed.) *In the Name of the Child. Health and Welfare 1880–1940*, 1992, pp. 45–71. Considers the medicalisation of the schoolchild against the backcloth of national efficiency concerns.

[103] F. Honigsbaum, 'The Interwar Health Insurance Scheme: a Rejoinder', in *Journal of Social Policy*, 12, 1983, 3, pp. 515–524. See also the Reply by N. Whiteside and M. Krafchik, pp. 525–529. The debate on causes of inadequate NHI provision. Honigsbaum targets the insurance societies, Whiteside [111] the lack of government commitment.

[104] P. Johnson, 'Social Risk and Social Welfare in Britain 1870–1939', *L.S.E. Working Papers in Economic History*, 3, 1992.

[105] J. Lewis and B. Brookes, 'The Peckham Health Centre, P.E.P. and the Concept of General Practice during the 1930s and 1940s', in *Medical Hist.*, 27, 1983, pp. 151–161.

[106] H. Marland, 'Lay and Medical conception of Medical Charity in the 19th century' in Barry and Jones (eds.) [95], pp. 149–171.

[107] C. Petty, 'The Medical Research Council's inter-war dietary surveys' in *Bulletin Soc. Hist. Med.*, 37, 1985, pp. 76–8. Evidence of medical attempt to blur direct links between poverty and ill-health. See forthcoming publications and [78].

[108] M. Powell, 'A Tale of Two Cities: A critical evaluation of the geographic provision of health care before the N.H.S.', in *Public Administration*, 70, 1992, 1, pp. 67–80. Suggests variations in interwar health care were not simply a function of wealthy or deprived geographical areas. See also [47].

[109] F. Prochaska, *Philanthropy and the Hospitals of London. The Kings Fund 1897–1990*, 1992. Important, but overstates the role of the Kings Fund and is atypical of hospital experience outside London.

[110] J.C. Riley, *Sickness, Recovery and Death: A History and Forecast of Ill Health*, 1989. Demonstrates the dangers of equating falling death rates with improving health levels.

[111] N. Whiteside, 'Private Agencies for Public Purposes: some new perspectives on policy making in Health Insurance between the wars', in *Journal of Social Policy*, 12, 1983, 2, pp. 165–194.

9 Contemporary sources cited in text

[112] J.S. Bristowe and T. Holmes, *Report on the Hospitals of the United Kingdom*, 6th *Report of the Medical Officer of the Privy Council*, 1863.

[113] H.C. Burdett, *Burdett's Hospitals and Charities*, 1889–1915.

[114] H.C. Burdett, *Burdett's Official Nursing Directory*, 1898.

[115] J.R and U.K. Hicks, Standards of Local Expenditure, *National Institute of Economic and Social Research Occasional Papers*, 3, 1943.

[116] Hospital Almoners Association, *Hospital Almoners Association Survey*, 1941.

[117] *Hospital and Health Review*, 1–39, 1921–24.

[118] *Hospital Gazette*, 1904–29.

[119] *Hospital Yearbook*, 1928–40.

[120] E.M. Hubback, *The Population of Britain*, 1947.

[121] Ministry of Health, *Annual Reports*, 1919–39.

[122] Ministry of Health, *Hospital Surveys*, 10 vols., 1945.

[123] G. Newman, *The Building of a Nation's Health*, 1939.

[124] A.Newsholme, *Medicine and the State*, 1932.

[125] PEP, *Report on British Health Services*, 1937.

[126] J.E. Stone, *Hospital Organisation and Management*, 1939.

[127] S. and B. Webb, *English Local Government, Vol.8. English Poor Law History, The Last Hundred Years*, Vol. I, 1929.

[128] S.and B. Webb, *The State and the Doctor*, 1910.

Addendum   A. Digby, *Making a medical living: doctors and their patients in the English market for medicine 1720–1911*, 1994.

Glossary

BHA	British Hospitals Association
BMA	British Medical Association
CDR	Crude Death Rate
CMO	Chief Medical Officer
EMS	Emergency Medical Service
GMC	General Medical Council
GP	General Practitioner
IMR	Infant Mortality Rate
LA	Local Authority
LCC	London County Council
LGB	Local Government Board
LSA	Licence of the Society of Apothecaries
MAB	Metropolitan Asylums Board
MMR	Maternal Mortality Rate
MoH, MosH	Medical Officer(s) of Health
Min of Health	Ministry of Health
NHI	National Health Insurance
PAC	Public Assistance Committee
PAI	Public Assistance Infirmary
RCN	Royal College of Nursing
RCP	Royal College of Physicians
STD	Sexually Transmitted Disease
RCS	Royal College of Surgeons
UDC	Urban District Council
VAD	Voluntary Aid Detachments

Index

(refers to sources cited in text: see also select bibliography)

USA, 6, 65

VD Act (1917), 55
Villiers, C., 44
Voluntary Aid Detachments, 37
voluntary effort, 70, 71
voluntary hospitals, 44–7, 60–1, 64
  access, 45, 64
  bed provision, 46, 47, 60
  childrens, 45
  exclusions, 8, 45
  finances, 46, 71–4
  London, 47, 61, 64, 71
  provincial, 47, 61
  Scottish, 46, 60, 72
  specialist, 45, 61
  subscriber-recommendation, 45,
    71, 73

World War One, 72
Voluntary Hospitals Council, 61,
  75

Webb, B., 51
Webster, C., 59
western bio medicine, 17
Whiteside, N., 70
Widows and Old Age Pensions Act,
  70
Wohl, A., 16
women doctors, 33, 50
women's health, 8, 25, 55, 58
works clubs, 42, 58
works collections, 72
World War One, 54

X-ray, 19

New Studies in Economic and Social History

Titles in the series available from Cambridge University Press:

Previously published as

Studies in Economic and Social History

Titles in the series available from the Macmillan Press Limited

1. B. W. E. Alford
    Depression and recovery? British economic growth, 1918–1939

2. M. Anderson
    Population change in north-western Europe, 1750–1850

3. S. D. Chapman
    The cotton industry in the industrial revolution: second edition

4. M. E. Falkus
    The industrialisation of Russia, 1700–1914

5. J. R. Harris
    The British iron industry, 1700–1850

6. J. Hatcher
    Plague, population and the English economy, 1348–1530

7. J. R. Hay
    The origins of the Liberal welfare reforms, 1906–1914

8. H. McLeod
    Religion and the working classes in nineteenth-century Britain

9. J. D. Marshall
    The Old Poor Law 1795–1834: second edition

10. R. J. Morris
    Class and class consciousness in the industrial revolution, 1750–1850

11. P. K. O'Brien
The economic effects of the American civil war

12. S. B. Saul
The myth of the Great Depression, 1873–1896: second edition

13. P. L. Payne
British entrepreneurship in the nineteenth century

14. G. C. Peden
Keynes, the treasury and British economic policy

15. M. E. Rose
The relief of poverty, 1834–1914

16. J. Thirsk
England's agricultural regions and agrarian history, 1500–1750

17. J. R. Ward
Poverty and progress in the Caribbean, 1800–1960

Economic History Society

The Economic History Society of Great Britain, which numbers around 3,000 members, publishes the *Economic History Review* four times a year (free to members) and holds an annual conference.

Enquiries about membership should be addressed to

The Assistant Secretary
Economic History Society
PO Box 70
Kingswood
Bristol
BS15 5TB

Full-time students may join at special rates.